The Carnivore's Gateway to Mediterranean Cuisine

Delicious Meals for Sworn Meat Lovers

By
Delia Bell

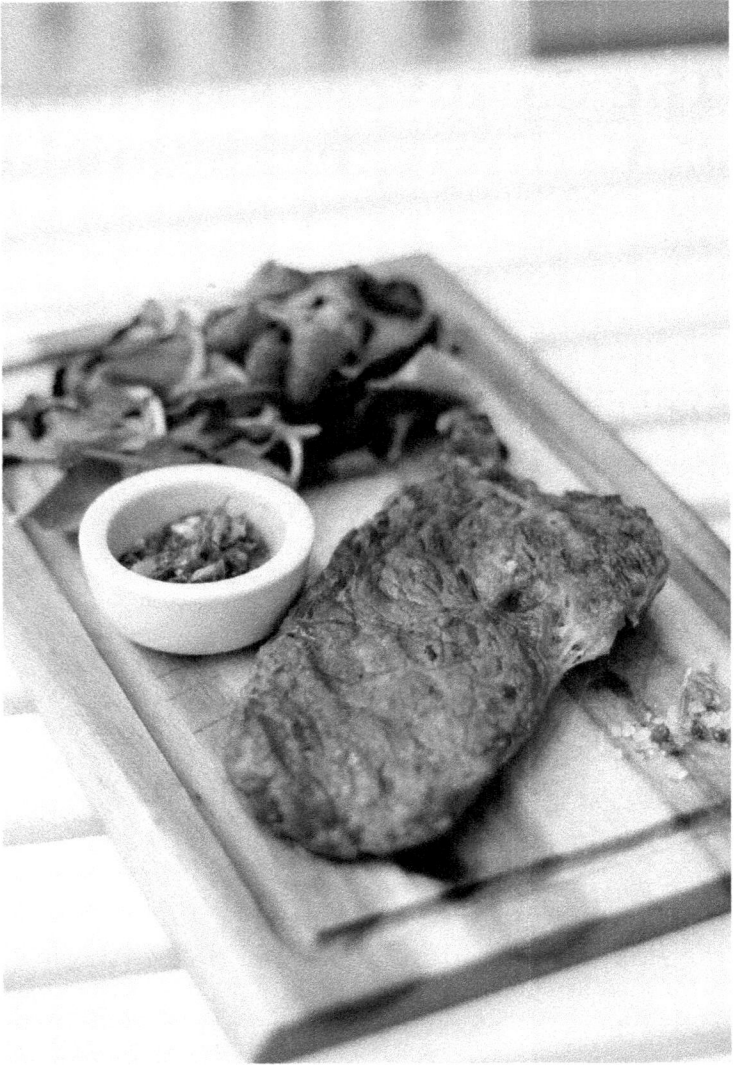

the publisher or the original author of this work can be in any fashion deemed liable for any hardship or damages that may befall them after undertaking information described herein.

Additionally, the information in the following pages is intended only for informational purposes and should thus be thought of as universal. As befitting its nature, it is presented without assurance regarding its prolonged validity or interim quality. Trademarks that are mentioned are done without written consent and can in no way be considered an endorsement from the trademark holder.

Table of Contents

INTRODUCTION

What is the Mediterranean Diet?

The Mediterranean diet is based on the diets of traditional eating habits from the 1960s of people from countries that surround the Mediterranean Sea, such as Greece, Italy, and Spain, and it encourages the consumption of fresh, seasonal, and local foods. The Mediterranean diet has become popular because individuals show low rates of heart disease, chronic disease, and obesity. The Mediterranean diet profile focuses on whole grains, good fats (fish, olive oil, nuts etc.), vegetables, fruits, fish, and very low consumption of any non-fish meat. Along with food, the Mediterranean diet emphasizes the need to spend time eating with family and physical activity. The Mediterranean diet is not a single prescribed diet, but rather a general food-based eating pattern, which is marked by local and cultural differences throughout the Mediterranean region.

The diet is generally characterized by a high intake of plant-based foods (e.g. fresh fruit and vegetables, nuts, and cereals) and olive oil, a moderate intake of fish and poultry, and low intakes of dairy products (mostly yoghurt and cheese), red and processed meats, and sweets. Wine is typically consumed in moderation and, normally, with a meal. A strong focus is placed on social and cultural aspects, such as communal mealtimes, resting after eating, and regular physical activity. Nowadays, however, the diet is no longer followed as widely as it was 30-50 years ago, as the diets of people living in these regions are becoming more 'Westernized' and higher in energy dense foods.

Benefits
The Mediterranean diet is not a weight loss, but increasing fiber intake and cutting out red meat, animal fats, and processed food may lead to weight loss. People who follow the diet may also have a lower risk of various diseases.

Heart health
In the 1950s,an American scientist, found that people living in the poorer areas of southern Italy had a lower risk of heart disease and death than those in wealthier parts of New York. Dr. Keys attributed this to diet. Since then, many studies have indicated that following a Mediterranean diet can help the body maintain healthy cholesterol levels and reduce the risk of high blood pressure and cardiovascular disease. The overall pattern of the Mediterranean diet is similar to their own dietary recommendations. A high proportion of calories on the diet come from fat, which can increase the risk of obesity. However, they also note that this fat is mainly unsaturated, which makes it a more healthful option than that from the typical American diet.

Protection from disease
The Mediterranean diet focuses on plant-based foods, and these are good sources of antioxidants.

The Mediterranean diet might offer protection from various cancers, and especially colorectal cancer. The reduction in risk may stem from the high intake of fruits, vegetables, and whole grains. By sticking to Mediterranean meals, people's levels of blood glucose and fats had decreased. During this time, there was also a lower incidence of stroke.

Diabetes

The Mediterranean diet may help prevent type 2 diabetes and improve markers of diabetes in people who already have the condition. Various other studies have concluded that following the Mediterranean diet can reduce the risk of type 2 diabetes and cardiovascular disease, which often occur together.

Food to eat

There is no single definition of the Mediterranean diet, but one group of scientists used the following as their 2015 basis of research.

Vegetables: Include 3 to 9 servings a day.

Fresh fruit: Up to 2 servings a day.

Cereals: Mostly whole grain from 1 to 13 servings a day.

Oil: Up to 8 servings of extra virgin (cold pressed) olive oil a day.

Fat — mostly unsaturated — made up 37% of the total calories. Unsaturated fat comes from plant sources, such as olives and avocado. The Mediterranean diet also provided 33 grams (g) of fiber a day. The baseline diet for this study provided around

2,200 calories a day. Typical ingredients. Here are some examples of ingredients that people often include in the Mediterranean diet.

Vegetables: Tomatoes, peppers, onions, eggplant, zucchini, cucumber, leafy green vegetables, plus others.
Fruits: Melon, apples, apricots, peaches, oranges, and lemons, and so on.
Legumes: Beans, lentils, and chickpeas.
Nuts and seeds: Almonds, walnuts, sunflower seeds, and cashews.
Unsaturated fat: Olive oil, sunflower oil, olives, and avocados.
Dairy products: Cheese and yogurt are the main dairy foods.
Cereals: These are mostly whole grain and include wheat and rice with bread accompanying many meals.
Fish: Sardines and other oily fish, as well as oysters and other shellfish. Poultry: Chicken or turkey.
Eggs: Chicken, quail, and duck eggs.
Drinks: A person can drink red wine in moderation.

The Mediterranean diet does not include strong liquor or carbonated and sweetened drinks. According to one definition, the diet limits red meat and sweets to less than 2 servings per week.

Food to avoid

Here's a list of foods you should generally limit while eating Mediterranean-style meals. Heavily processed foods. Let's be real: Many, many foods are processed to some degree. A can of beans has been processed, in the sense that the beans have been cooked before being canned. Olive oil has been processed, because olives have been turned into oil. But when we talk about limiting processed foods, this really means avoiding things like frozen meals with tons of sodium. You should also limit soda, desserts and candy. As the adage goes, if the ingredient list includes items that your great-grandparents wouldn't recognize as food, it's probably processed. If you're buying a packaged food that's as close to its whole-food form as possible — such as frozen fruit or veggies with nothing added — you're good to go.

Processed red meat

On the Mediterranean diet, you should minimize your intake of red meat, such as steak. What about processed red meat, such as hot dogs and bacon? You should avoid these foods or limit them as much as possible. A study published in BMJ found that regularly eating red meat, especially processed varieties, was associated with a higher risk of death. Butter. Here's another food that should be limited on the Mediterranean diet. Use olive oil instead, which has many heart health benefits and contains less saturated fat than butter. According to the USDA National Nutrient Database, butter has 7 grams of saturated fat per tablespoon, while olive oil has about 2 grams.

Refined grains

The Mediterranean diet is centered around whole grains, such as farro, millet, couscous and brown rice. With this eating style, you'll generally want to limit your intake of refined grains such as white pasta and white bread.

Alcohol

When you're following the Mediterranean diet, red wine should be your chosen alcoholic drink. This is because red wine offers health benefits, particularly for the heart. But it's important to limit intake of any type of alcohol to up to one drink per day for women, as well as men older than 65, and up to two drinks daily for men age 65 and younger. The amount that counts as a drink is 5 ounces of wine, 12 ounces of beer or 1.5 ounces of 80-proof liquor.

Yummy Turkey Meatballs

Servings: 4

Cooking Time: 25 Minutes

Ingredients:

- ¼ yellow onion, finely diced
- 1 14-oz can of artichoke hearts, diced
- 1 lb. ground turkey
- 1 tsp dried parsley
- 1 tsp oil
- 4 tbsp fresh basil, finely chopped
- Pepper and salt to taste

Directions:

1. Grease a cookie sheet and preheat oven to 3500F.

2. On medium fire, place a nonstick medium saucepan and sauté artichoke hearts and diced onions for 5 minutes or until onions are soft.

3. Remove from fire and let cool.

4. Meanwhile, in a big bowl, mix with hands parsley, basil and ground turkey. Season to taste.

5. Once onion mixture has cooled add into the bowl and mix thoroughly.

6. With an ice cream scooper, scoop ground turkey and form into balls, makes around 6 balls.

7. Place on prepped cookie sheet, pop in the oven and bake until cooked through around 15-20 minutes.

8. Remove from pan, serve and enjoy.

Nutrition Info: Calories per Serving: 328; Carbs: 11.8g; Protein: 33.5g; Fat: 16.3g

Garlic Caper Beef Roast

Servings: 4
Cooking Time: 40 Minutes

Ingredients:
- 2 lbs beef roast, cubed
- 1 tbsp fresh parsley, chopped
- 1 tbsp capers, chopped
- 1 tbsp garlic, minced
- 1 cup chicken stock
- 1/2 tsp dried rosemary
- 1/2 tsp ground cumin
- 1 onion, chopped
- 1 tbsp olive oil
- Pepper
- Salt

Directions:
1. Add oil into the instant pot and set the pot on sauté mode.
2. Add garlic and onion and sauté for 5 minutes.
3. Add meat and cook until brown.
4. Add remaining ingredients and stir well.
5. Seal pot with lid and cook on high for 30 minutes.
6. Once done, allow to release pressure naturally. Remove lid.

7. Stir well and serve.

Nutrition Info: Calories 470 Fat 17.9 g Carbohydrates 3.9 g Sugar 1.4 g Protein 69.5 g Cholesterol 203 mg

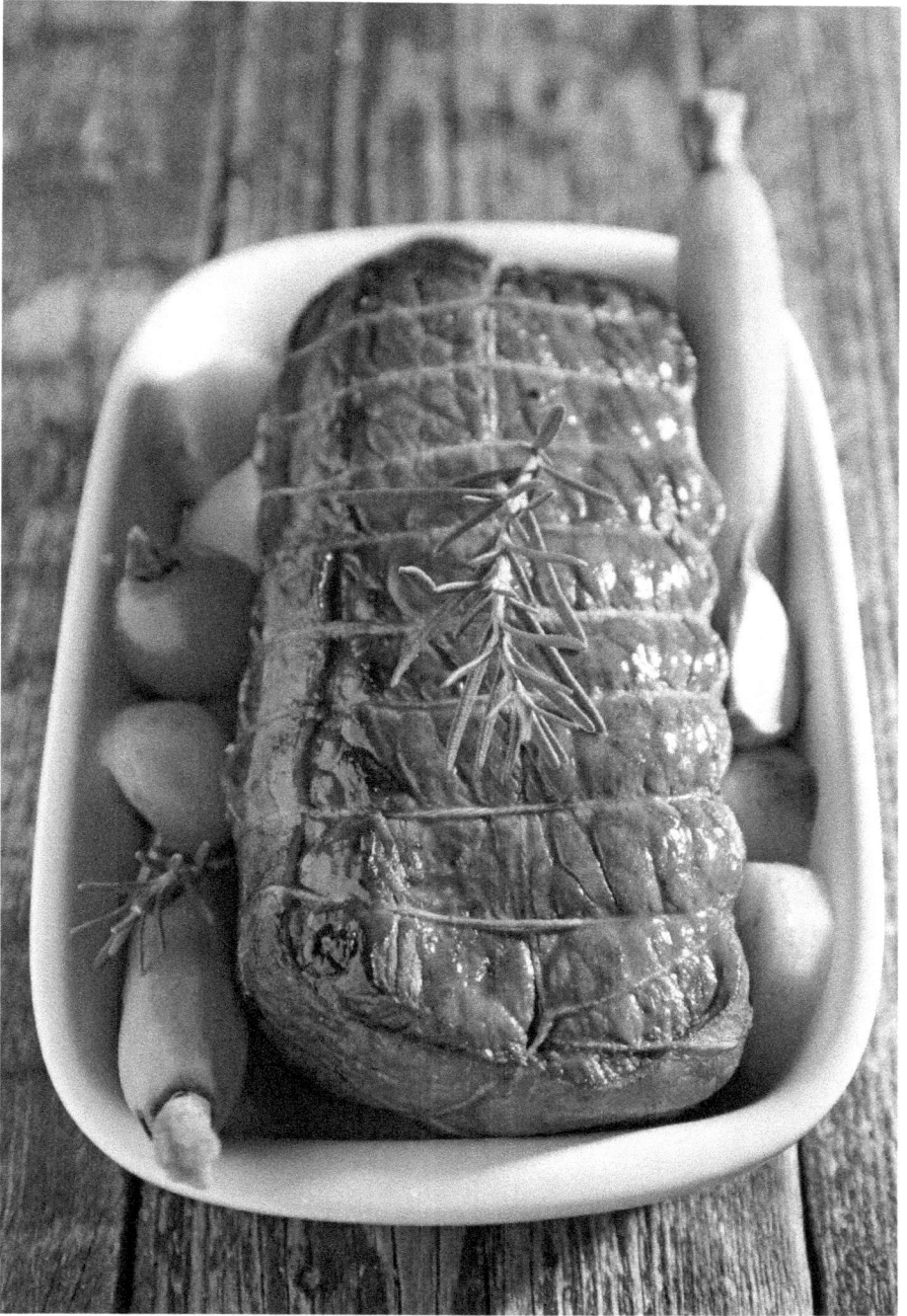

Olive Oil Drenched Lemon Chicken

Servings: 4

Cooking Time: 60 Minutes

Ingredients:
- 1 lemon, thinly sliced
- 1 red bell pepper, cut into 1-inch wide strips
- 1 red onion, cut into 1-inch wedges
- 1 tablespoon dried oregano
- 1/2 teaspoon coarsely ground black pepper
- 1/4 cup olive oil
- 2 tablespoons fresh lemon juice
- 2 tablespoons fresh lemon zest
- 3/4 teaspoon salt
- 4 large cloves garlic, pressed
- 4 skinless, boneless chicken breast halves
- 8 baby red potatoes, halved

Directions:

1. Preheat oven to 400oF.

2. In a bowl, mix well pepper, salt, oregano, garlic, lemon zest, lemon juice, and olive oil.

3. In a 9 x 13-inch casserole dish, evenly spread chicken in a single layer. Brush lemon juice mixture over chicken.

4. In a bowl mix well lemon slices, red onion, bell pepper, and potatoes. Drizzle remaining olive oil sauce and toss

well to coat. Arrange vegetables and lemon slices around chicken breasts in baking dish.

5. Bake for 50 minutes; brush chicken and vegetables with pan drippings halfway through cooking time.

6. Let chicken rest for ten minutes before serving.

Nutrition Info: Calories per Serving: 517; Carbs: 65.1g; Protein: 30.8g; Fats: 16.7g

Beef Spread

Servings: 4

Cooking Time: 25 Minutes

Ingredients:
- 8 oz beef liver
- ½ onion, peeled
- ½ carrot, peeled
- ½ teaspoon peppercorns
- 1 bay leaf
- ½ teaspoon salt
- 1/3 cup water
- 1 teaspoon ground black pepper

Directions:

1. Chop the beef liver and put it in the saucepan.

2. Add onion, carrot, peppercorns, bay leaf, salt, and ground black pepper.

3. Add water and close the lid.

4. Boil the beef liver for 25 minutes or until all ingredients are tender.

5. Transfer the cooked mixture in the blender and blend it until smooth.

6. Then place the cooked pate in the serving bowl and flatten the surface of it.

7. Refrigerate the pate for 20-30 minutes before serving.

Nutrition Info:Per Serving:calories 109, fat 2.7, fiber 0.6, carbs 5.3, protein 15.3

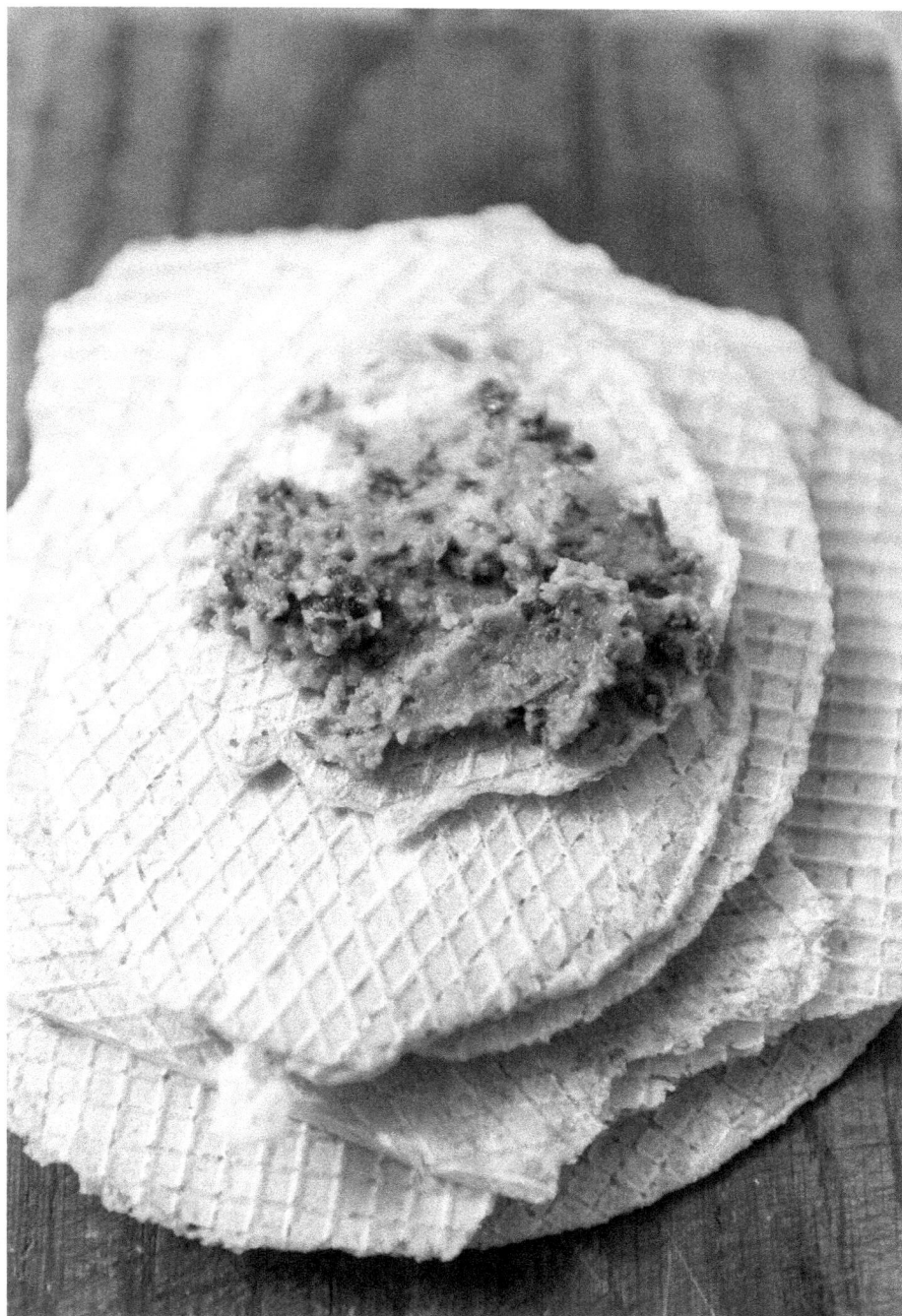

Pork Chops And Relish

Servings: 6
Cooking Time: 14 Minutes

Ingredients:
- 6 pork chops, boneless
- 7 ounces marinated artichoke hearts, chopped and their liquid reserved A pinch of salt and black pepper
- 1 teaspoon hot pepper sauce
- 1 and ½ cups tomatoes, cubed
- 1 jalapeno pepper, chopped
- ½ cup roasted bell peppers, chopped
- ½ cup black olives, pitted and sliced

Directions:
1. In a bowl, mix the chops with the pepper sauce, reserved liquid from the artichokes, cover and keep in the fridge for 15 minutes.
2. Heat up a grill over medium-high heat, add the pork chops and cook for 7 minutes on each side.
3. In a bowl, combine the artichokes with the peppers and the remaining ingredients, toss, divide on top of the chops and serve.

Nutrition Info: calories 215, fat 6, fiber 1, carbs 6, protein 35

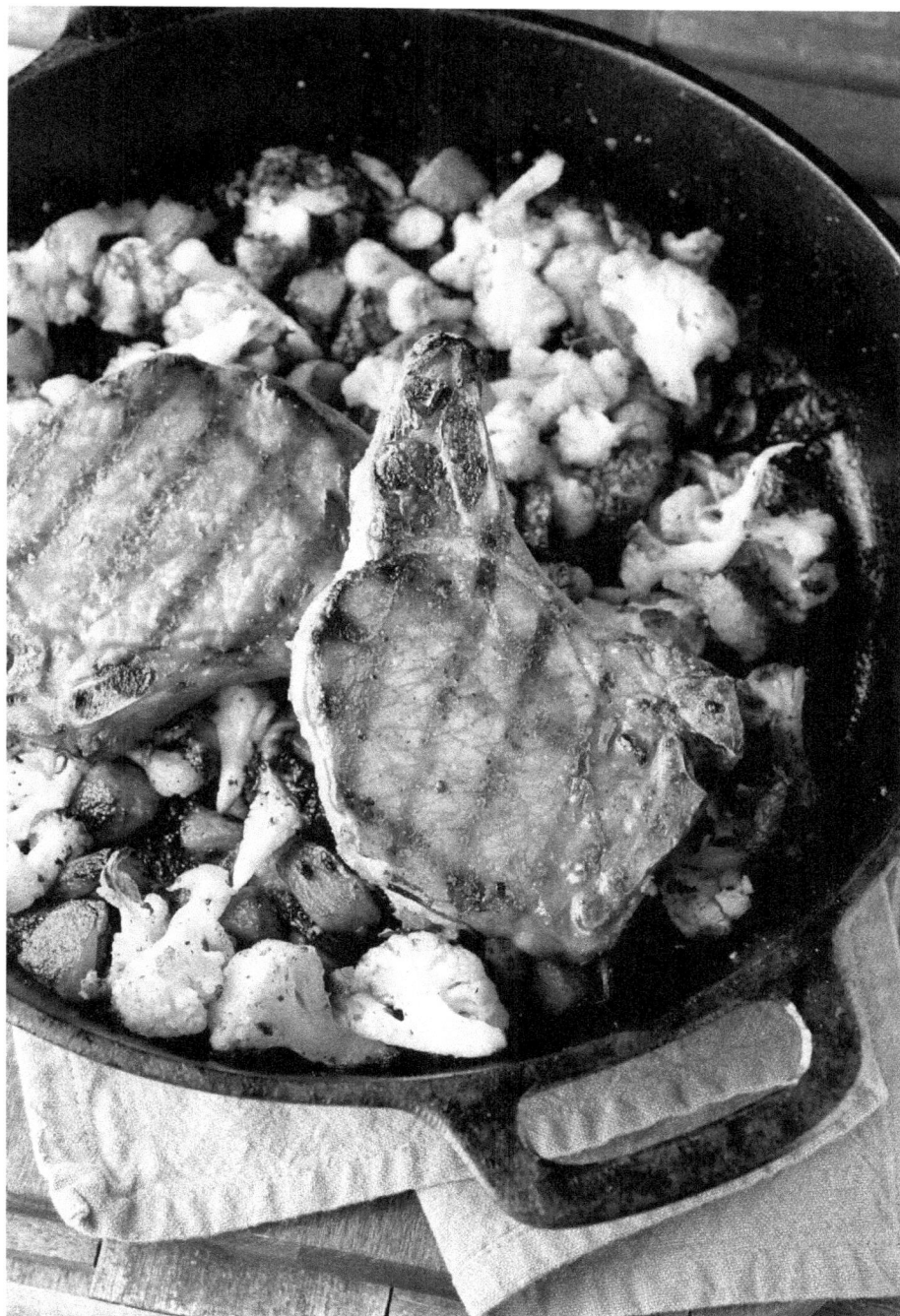

Tasty Beef Goulash

Servings: 2

Cooking Time: 30 Minutes

Ingredients:

- 1/2 lb beef stew meat, cubed
- 1 tbsp olive oil
- 1/2 onion, chopped
- 1/2 cup sun-dried tomatoes, chopped
- 1/4 zucchini, chopped
- 1/2 cabbage, sliced
- 1 1/2 tbsp olive oil
- 2 cups chicken broth
- Pepper
- Salt

Directions:

1. Add oil into the instant pot and set the pot on sauté mode.
2. Add onion and sauté for 3-5 minutes.
3. Add tomatoes and cook for 5 minutes.
4. Add remaining ingredients and stir well.
5. Seal pot with lid and cook on high for 20 minutes.
6. Once done, allow to release pressure naturally for 10 minutes then release remaining using quick release. Remove lid.

7. Stir well and serve.

Nutrition Info: Calories 389 Fat 15.8 g Carbohydrates 19.3 g Sugar 10.7 g Protein 43.2 g Cholesterol 101 mg

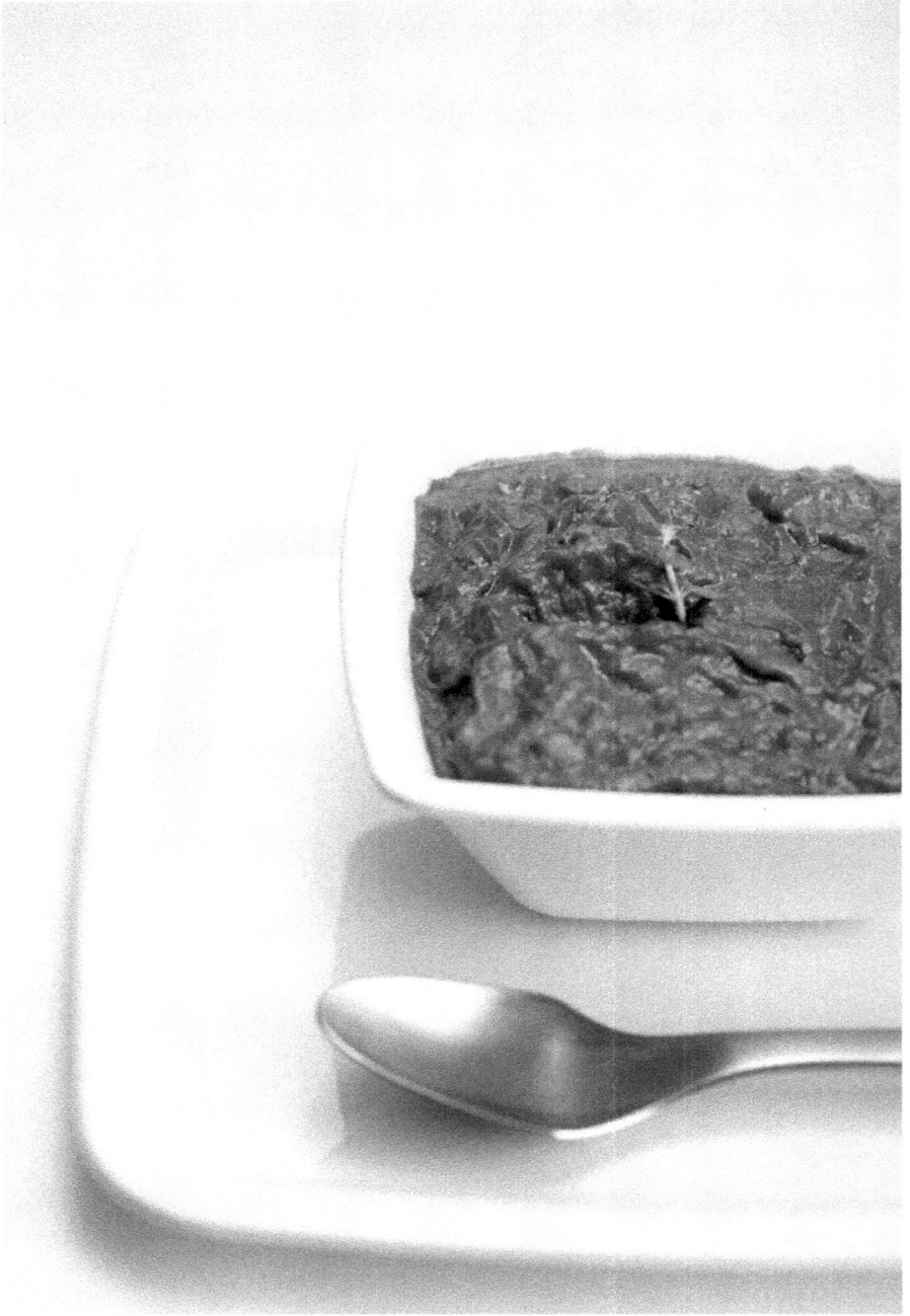

Beef And Grape Sauce

Servings: 4

Cooking Time: 25 Minutes

Ingredients:

- 1-pound beef sirloin
- 1 teaspoon molasses
- 1 tablespoon lemon zest, grated
- 1 teaspoon soy sauce
- 1 chili pepper, chopped
- ¼ teaspoon fresh ginger, minced
- 1 cup grape juice
- ½ teaspoon salt
- 1 tablespoon butter

Directions:

1. Sprinkle the beef sirloin with salt and minced ginger.

2. Heat up butter in the saucepan and add meat.

3. Roast it for 5 minutes from each side over the medium heat.

4. After this, add soy sauce, chili pepper, and grape juice.

5. Then add lemon zest and simmer the meat for 10 minutes.

6. Add molasses and mix up meat well.

7. Close the lid and cook meat for 5 minutes.

8. Serve the cooked beef with grape juice sauce.

Nutrition Info:Per Serving:calories 267, fat 10, fiber 0.2, carbs 7.4, protein 34.9

Lamb And Tomato Sauce

Servings: 3
Cooking Time: 55 Minutes

Ingredients:
- 9 oz lamb shanks
- 1 onion, diced
- 1 carrot, diced
- 1 tablespoon olive oil
- 1 teaspoon salt
- 1 teaspoon ground black pepper
- 1 ½ cup chicken stock
- 1 tablespoon tomato paste

Directions:
1. Sprinkle the lamb shanks with salt and ground black pepper.
2. Heat up olive oil in the saucepan.
3. Add lamb shanks and roast them for 5 minutes from each side.
4. Transfer meat in the plate.
5. After this, add onion and carrot in the saucepan.
6. Roast the vegetables for 3 minutes.
7. Add tomato paste and mix up well.
8. Then add chicken stock and bring the liquid to boil.
9. Add lamb shanks, stir well, and close the lid.

10. Cook the meat for 40 minutes over the medium-low heat.

Nutrition Info:Per Serving:calories 232, fat 11.3, fiber 1.7, carbs 7.3, protein 25.1

Lamb And Sweet Onion Sauce

Servings: 4
Cooking Time: 40 Minutes

Ingredients:

- 2 pounds lamb meat, cubed
- 1 tablespoon sweet paprika
- Salt and black pepper to the taste
- 1 and ½ cups veggie stock
- 4 garlic cloves, minced
- 2 tablespoons olive oil
- 1 pound sweet onion, chopped
- 1 cup balsamic vinegar

Directions:
1. Heat up a pot with the oil over medium heat, add the onion, vinegar, salt and pepper, stir and cook for 10 minutes.
2. Add the meat and the rest of the ingredients, toss, bring to a simmer and cook over medium heat for 30 minutes.
3. Divide the mix between plates and serve.

Nutrition Info: calories 303, fat 12.3, fiber 7.1, carbs 15.2, protein 17.0

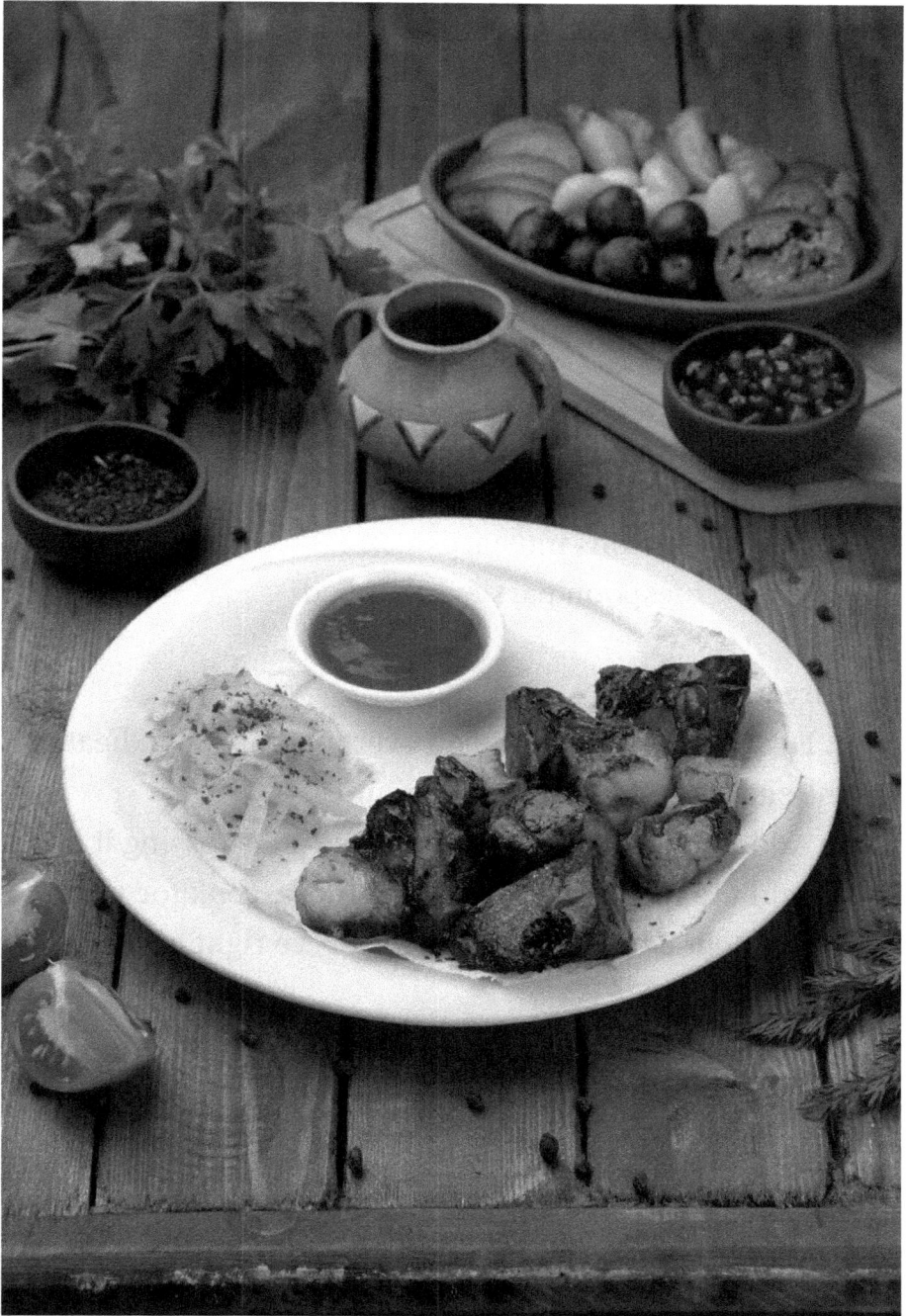

Pork And Mustard Shallots Mix

Servings: 4

Cooking Time: 25 Minutes

Ingredients:

- 3 shallots, chopped
- 1 pound pork loin, cut into strips
- ½ cup veggie stock
- 2 tablespoons olive oil
- A pinch of salt and black pepper
- 2 teaspoons mustard
- 1 tablespoon parsley, chopped

Directions:

1. Heat up a pan with the oil over medium-high heat, add the shallots and sauté for 5 minutes.

2. Add the meat and cook for 10 minutes tossing it often.

3. Add the rest of the ingredients, toss, cook for 10 minutes more, divide between plates and serve right away.

Nutrition Info: calories 296, fat 12.4, fiber 9.3, carbs 13.5, protein 22.5

Rosemary Lamb

Servings: 4

Cooking Time: 6 Hours

Ingredients:

- 2 pounds lamb shoulder, cubed
- 1 tablespoon rosemary, chopped
- 3 garlic cloves, minced
- ½ cup lamb stock
- 4 bay leaves
- Salt and black pepper to the taste

Directions:

1. In your slow cooker, combine the lamb with the rosemary and the rest of the ingredients, put the lid on and cook on High for 6 hours.
2. Divide the mix between palates and serve.

Nutrition Info: calories 292, fat 13.2, fiber 11.6, carbs 18.3, protein 14.2

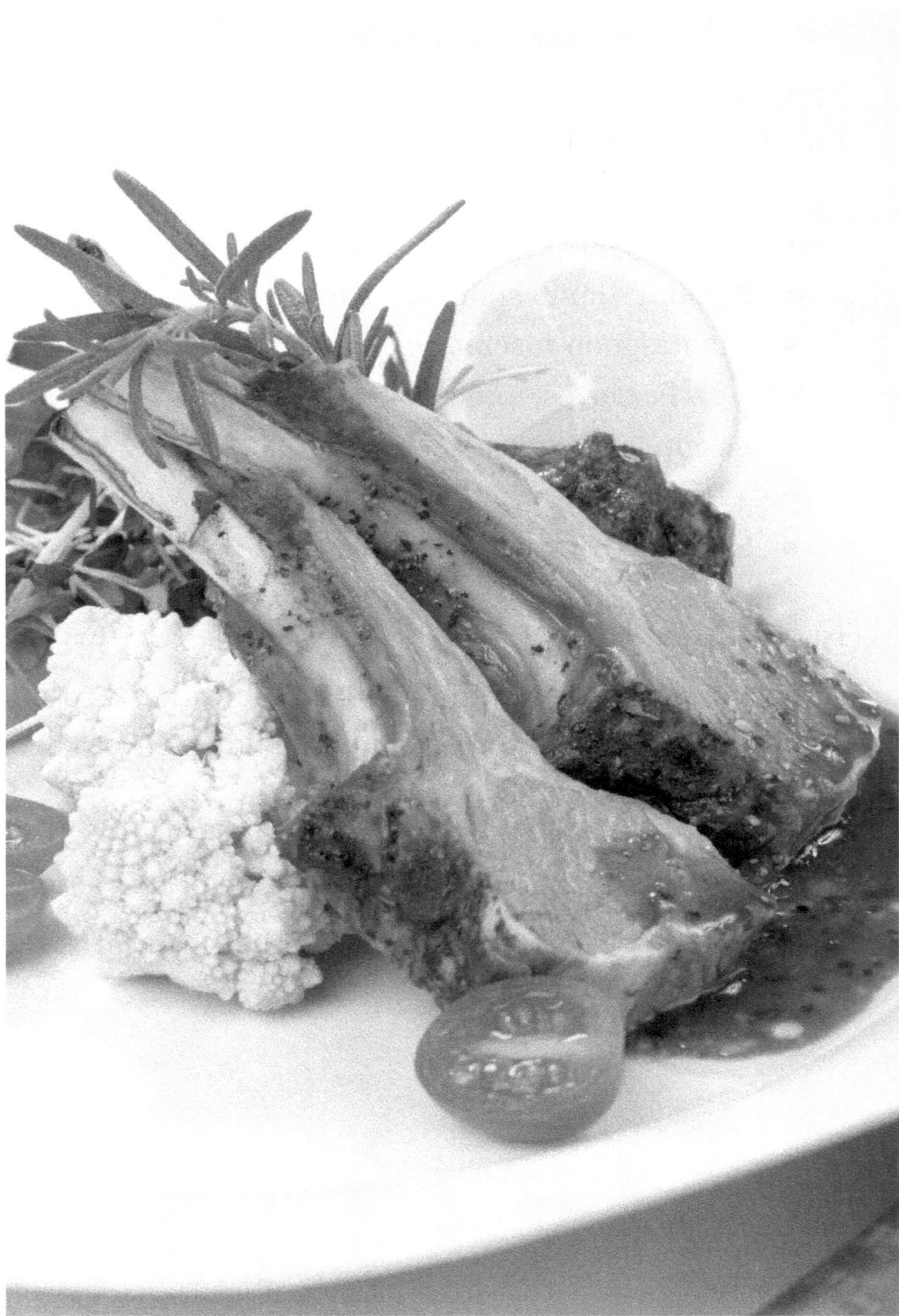

Mouth-watering Lamb Stew

Servings: 4
Cooking Time: 180 Minutes

Ingredients:
- ½ cup golden raisins
- 1 cup dates, cut in half
- 1 cup dried figs, cut in half
- 1 lb. lamb shoulder, trimmed of fat and cut into 2-inch cubes 1 onion, minced
- 1 tbsp fresh coriander, roughly chopped
- 1 tbsp honey, optional
- 1 tbsp olive oil
- 1 tbsp Ras el Hanout
- 2 cloves garlic, minced
- 2 cups beef stock or lamb stock
- Pepper and salt to taste
- ¼ tsp ground cloves
- ½ tsp ground black pepper
- 1 tsp ground turmeric
- 1 tsp ground nutmeg
- 1 tsp ground allspice
- 1 tsp ground cinnamon
- 2 tsp ground mace
- 2 tsp ground cardamom
- 2 tsp ground ginger
- ½ tsp anise seeds'1/2 tsp ground cayenne pepper

Directions:

1. Preheat oven to 300F.

2. In small bowl, add all Ras el Hanout ingredients and mix thoroughly. Just get what the ingredients need and store remaining in a tightly lidded spice jar.

3. On high fire, place a heavy bottomed medium pot and heat olive oil. Once hot, brown lamb pieces on each side for around 3 to 4 minutes.

4. Lower fire to medium high and add remaining ingredients, except for the coriander.

5. Mix well. Season with pepper and salt to taste. Cover pot and bring to a boil.

6. Once boiling, turn off fire, and pop pot into oven.

7. Bake uncovered for 2 to 2.5 hours or until meat is fork tender.

8. Once meat is tender, remove from oven.

9. To serve, sprinkle fresh coriander, and enjoy.

Nutrition Info: Calories per Serving: 633.4; Carbs: 78.1g; Protein: 33.0g; Fat: 21.0g

Beef With Tomatoes

Servings: 4
Cooking Time: 40 Minutes

Ingredients:

- 2 lb beef roast, sliced
- 1 tbsp chives, chopped
- 1 tsp garlic, minced
- 1/2 tsp chili powder
- 2 tbsp olive oil
- 1 onion, chopped
- 1 cup beef stock
- 1 tbsp oregano, chopped
- 1 cup tomatoes, chopped
- Pepper
- Salt

Directions:

1. Add oil into the instant pot and set the pot on sauté mode.

2. Add garlic, onion, and chili powder and sauté for 5 minutes.

3. Add meat and cook for 5 minutes.

4. Add remaining ingredients and stir well.

5. Seal pot with lid and cook on high for 30 minutes.

6. Once done, allow to release pressure naturally for 10 minutes then release remaining using quick release. Remove lid.

7. Stir well and serve.

Nutrition Info: Calories 511 Fat 21.6 g Carbohydrates 5.6 g Sugar 2.5 g Protein 70.4 g Cholesterol 203 mg

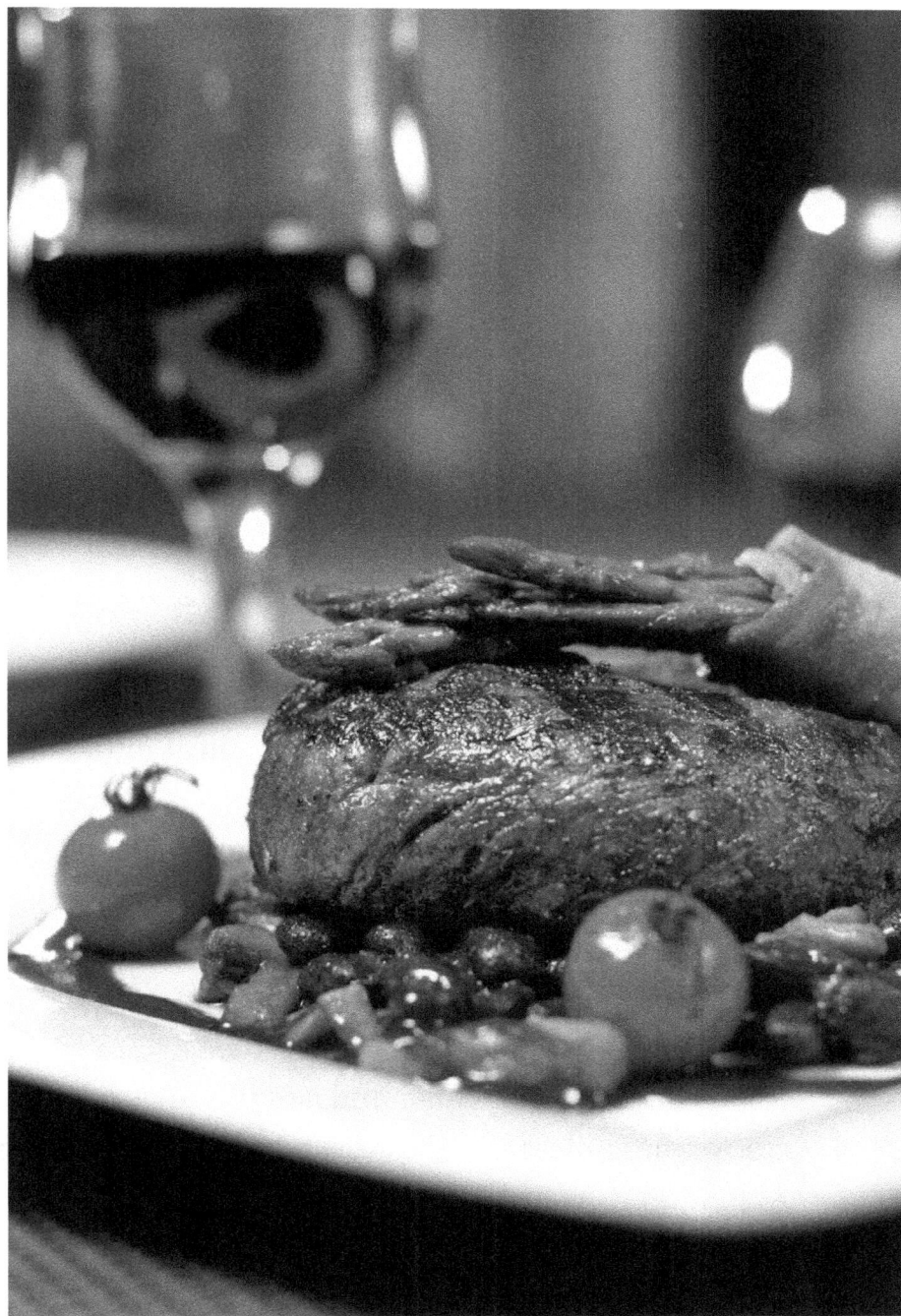

Chicken Thighs With Butternut Squash

Servings: 6

Cooking Time: 30 Minutes

Ingredients:

- ½ pound bacon
- 3 cups butternut squash, cubed
- 6 boneless chicken thighs
- A sprig of fresh sage, chopped
- Extra coconut oil for frying
- Salt and pepper to taste

Directions:

1. Preheat the oven to 425F.

2. In a skillet, fry the bacon over medium heat until crisp. Set aside then crumble.

3. In the same skillet, sauté the butternut squash and season with salt and pepper to taste. Once the squash is cooked, remove from the skillet and set aside.

4. Using the same skillet, add coconut oil and cook the chicken thighs for 10 minutes on each side.

5. Season with salt and pepper and add the squash back.

6. Remove the skillet from the stove and bake in the oven for 15 minutes. 7. Garnish with bacon.

Nutrition Info: Calories per Serving: 315.3; Carbs: 11.3g; Protein: 25.0g; Fat: 18.9g

Lamb And Peanuts Mix

Servings: 4

Cooking Time: 20 Minutes

Ingredients:

- 2 tablespoons lime juice
- 1 tablespoon balsamic vinegar
- 5 garlic cloves, minced
- 2 tablespoons olive oil
- Salt and black pepper to the taste
- 1 and ½ pound lamb meat, cubed
- 3 tablespoons peanuts, toasted and chopped
- 2 scallions, chopped

Directions:

1. Heat up a pan with the oil over medium-high heat, add the meat, and
cook for 4 minutes on each side.

2. Add the scallions and the garlic and sauté for 2 minutes more.

3. Add the rest of the ingredients, toss cook for 10 minutes more, divide between plates and serve right away.

Nutrition Info: calories 300, fat 14.5, fiber 9.1, carbs 15.7, protein 17.5

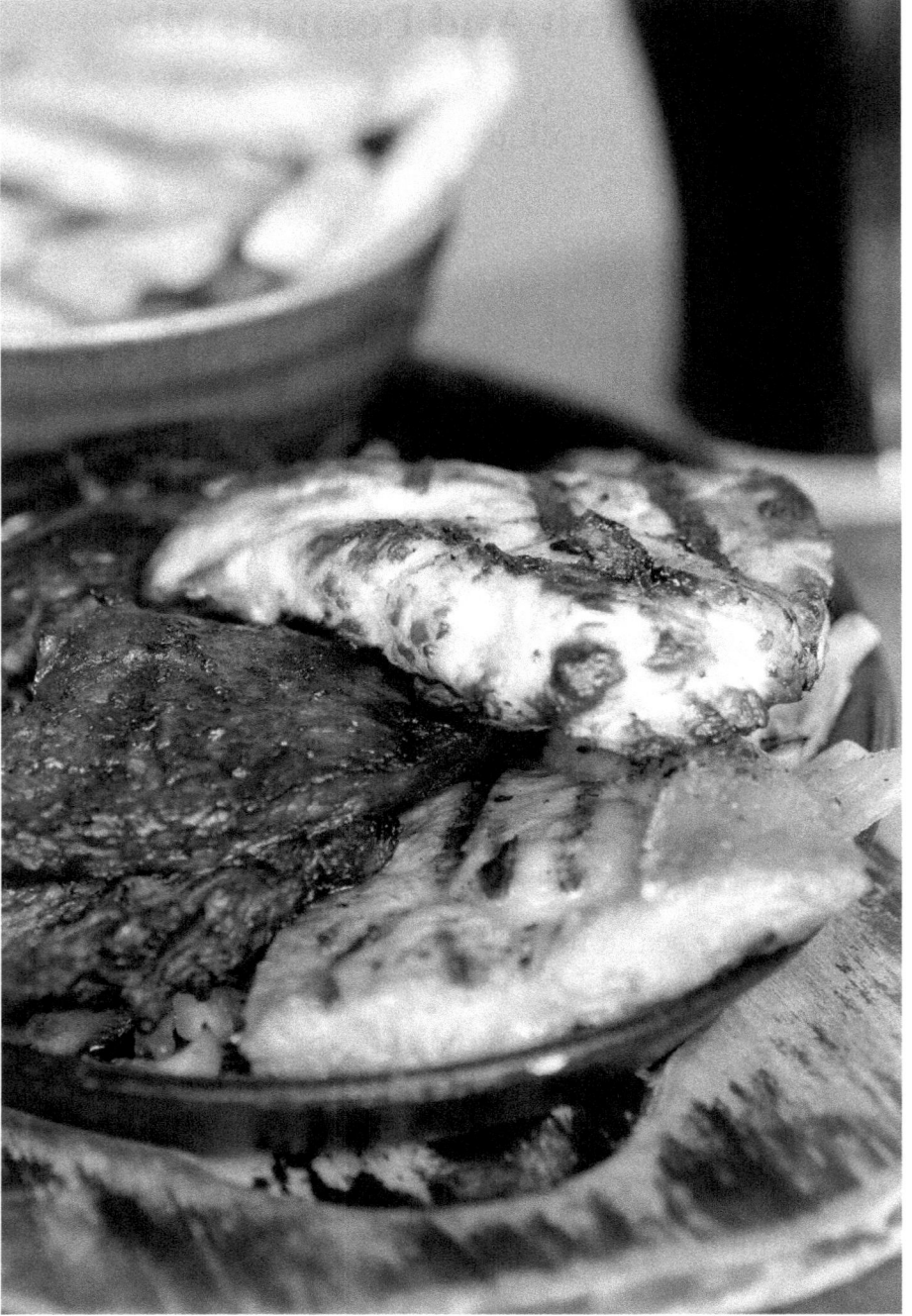

Grilled Chicken Breasts

Servings: 4
Cooking Time: 15 Minutes

Ingredients:
- 4 boneless skinless chicken breast halves
- 3 tablespoons lemon juice
- 3 tablespoons olive oil
- 3 tablespoons chopped fresh parsley
- 3 garlic cloves, crushed and minced
- 1 teaspoon paprika
- 1⁄2 teaspoon dried oregano
- 1/2 teaspoon salt
- 1/2 teaspoon pepper

Directions:
1. In a large Ziplock bag, mix well oregano, paprika, garlic, parsley, olive oil, and lemon juice.
2. Pierce chicken with knife several times and sprinkle with salt and pepper.
3. Add chicken to bag and marinate 20 minutes or up to two days in the fridge.
4. Remove chicken from bag and grill for 5 minutes per side in a 3500F preheated grill.
5. Remove chicken from grill and let it stand on a plate for 5 minutes before slicing.

6. Serve and enjoy with a side of rice or salad.

Nutrition Info: Calories per Serving: 485; Carbs: 2.7g; Protein: 72.8g; Fats: 19.3g

Grilled Veggies And Chicken

Servings: 3

Cooking Time: 20 Minutes

Ingredients:

- ¼ teaspoon cayenne pepper
- ½ teaspoon garlic granules
- ½ teaspoon onion powder
- 1 cup organic tomatoes, blended
- 1 red onion
- 1 red pepper, chopped
- 1 tablespoon vinegar
- 1 teaspoon Italian seasoning
- 1 teaspoon rosemary
- 1 yellow squash, chopped
- 1 zucchini, chopped
- 1-pound organic chicken breast
- 2 cups fresh cherry tomatoes, halved
- 4 tablespoon extra-virgin olive oil
- Pepper to taste
- Salt to taste

Directions:

1. Marinade the chicken by mixing together 1 tablespoon of extra virgin olive oil, Italian seasoning, and rosemary. Season with salt and set aside for at least 2 hours.

2. In another bowl, make the salad by combining the red onion, fresh cherry tomatoes, red pepper, squash and zucchini. Add 1 tablespoon of extra virgin olive oil and season with salt and pepper to taste. Place inside a greased tin foil then set aside.

3. Prepare the grill and heat it to 350F. Cook the chicken breast and let it cook for 7 minutes on each side. Place the tinfoil with the veggies on the grill and cook it for five to 7 minutes.

4. Meanwhile, make the vinaigrette by combining the cayenne pepper, onion powder, garlic granules, vinegar and blended organic tomatoes in a food processor. Add 2 tablespoon of extra virgin olive oil and season with salt and pepper to taste.

Nutrition Info: Calories per Serving: 363.6; Carbs: 14.2g; Protein: 45.2g; Fat:

14.0g

Oregano-smoked Paprika Baked Chicken

Servings: 2

Cooking Time: 40 Minutes

Ingredients:
- 1 tbsp dried oregano
- 1 tsp freshly ground black pepper
- 1 tsp Himalayan salt
- 1 tsp smoked paprika
- 2 green onions, sliced
- 2 jalapeño peppers, seeded and sliced
- 2 large boneless, skinless chicken breasts (about 400g/14oz each) 2 medium tomatoes, diced
- 6 mini bell peppers of assorted colors, seeded and chopped
- The juice of 1 lime

Directions:

1. Preheat oven to 450°F.

2. Mix all the spices in a small bowl. Rub all over chicken breasts.

3. Lightly grease an oven-proof dish with olive oil.

4. Place the chicken breasts in the dish and arrange the vegetables around it.

5. Cover with aluminum foil and bake for 35 minutes.

6. Set the oven to broil, remove the foil and cook under the broiler about 5 minutes, or until the chicken becomes golden brown.

7. Let the chicken rest for 5 minutes before slicing and serving.

Nutrition Info: Calories per Serving: 286; Carbs: 14.1g; Protein: 45.1g; Fats: 5.5g

Cheddar Lamb And Zucchinis

Servings: 4

Cooking Time: 30 Minutes

Ingredients:

- 1 pound lamb meat, cubed
- 1 tablespoon avocado oil
- 2 cups zucchinis, chopped
- ½ cup red onion, chopped
- Salt and black pepper to the taste
- 15 ounces canned roasted tomatoes, crushed
- ¾ cup cheddar cheese, shredded

Directions:

1. Heat up a pan with the oil over medium-high heat, add the meat and the onion and brown for 5 minutes.

2. Add the rest of the ingredients except the cheese, bring to a simmer and cook over medium heat for 20 minutes.

3. Add the cheese, cook everything for 5 minutes more, divide between plates and serve.

Nutrition Info: calories 306, fat 16.4, fiber 12.3, carbs 15.5, protein 18.5

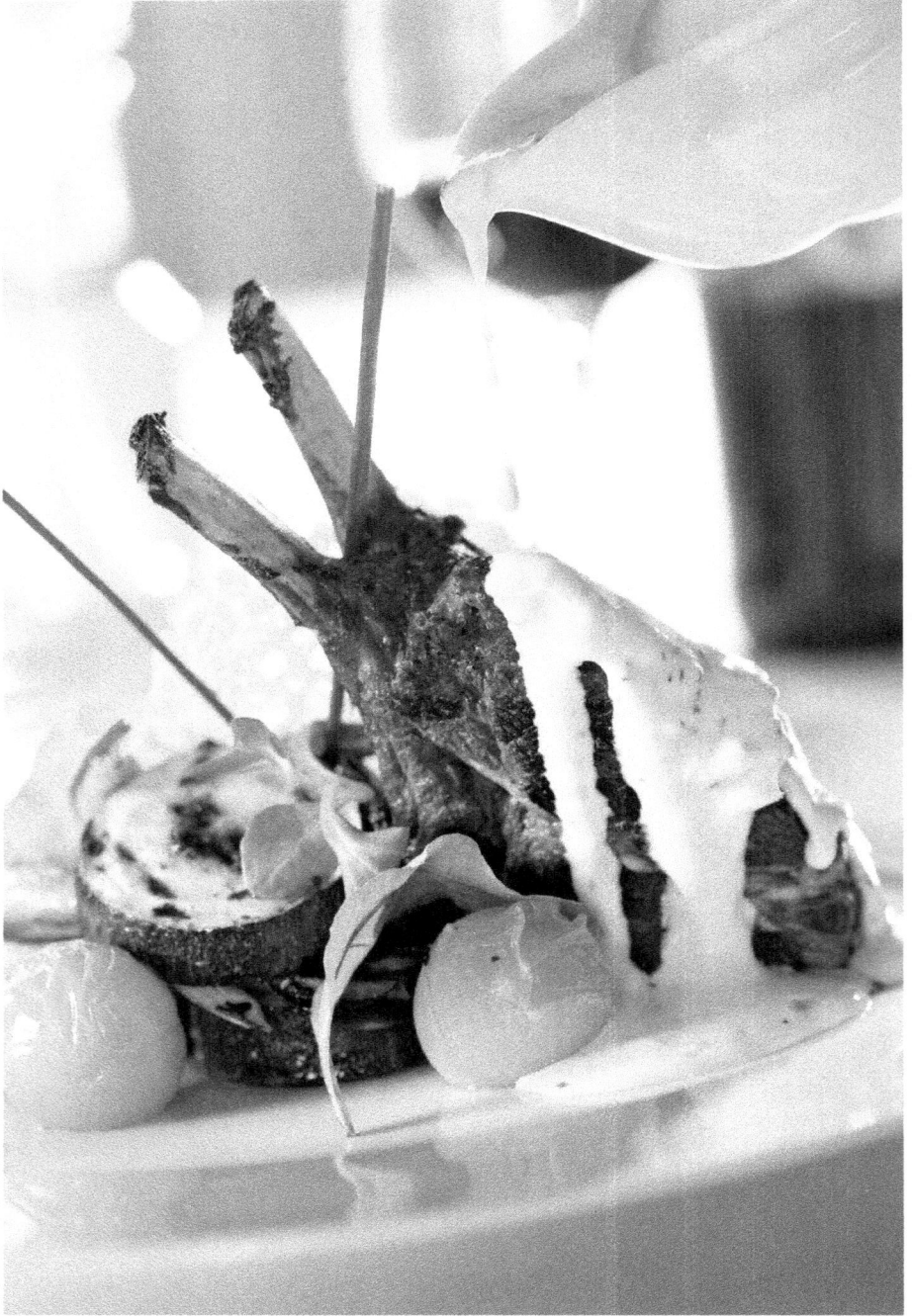

Fennel Pork

Servings: 4

Cooking Time: 2 Hours

Ingredients:

- 2 pork loin roast, trimmed, and boneless
- Salt and black pepper to the taste
- 3 garlic cloves, minced
- 2 teaspoons fennel, ground
- 1 tablespoon fennel seeds
- 2 teaspoons red pepper, crushed
- ¼ cup olive oil

Directions:

1. In a roasting pan, combine the pork with salt, pepper and the rest of the ingredients, toss, introduce in the oven and bake at 380 degrees F for 2 hours.

2. Slice the roast, divide between plates and serve with a side salad.

Nutrition Info: calories 300, fat 4, fiber 2, carbs 6, protein 15

Lamb And Feta Artichokes

Servings: 6

Cooking Time: 8 Hours And 5 Minutes

Ingredients:

- 2 pounds lamb shoulder, boneless and roughly cubed
- 2 spring onions, chopped
- 1 tablespoon olive oil
- 3 garlic cloves, minced
- 1 tablespoon lemon juice
- Salt and black pepper to the taste
- 1 and ½ cups veggie stock
- 6 ounces canned artichoke hearts, drained and quartered
- ½ cup feta cheese, crumbled
- 2 tablespoons parsley, chopped

Directions:

1. Heat up a pan with the oil over medium-high heat, add the lamb, brown 5 minutes and transfer to your slow cooker.

2. Add the rest of the ingredients except the parsley and the cheese, put the lid on and cook on Low for 8 hours.

3. Add the cheese and the parsley, divide the mix between plates and serve.

Nutrition Info: calories 330, fat 14.5, fiber 14.1, carbs 21.7, protein 17.5

Lamb And Plums Mix

Servings: 4

Cooking Time: 6 Hours And 10 Minutes

Ingredients:

- 4 lamb shanks
- 1 red onion, chopped
- 2 tablespoons olive oil
- 1 cup plums, pitted and halved
- 1 tablespoon sweet paprika
- 2 cups chicken stock
- Salt and pepper to the taste

Directions:

1. Heat up a pan with the oil over medium-high heat, add the lamb, brown for 5 minutes on each side and transfer to your slow cooker.

2. Add the rest of the ingredients, put the lid on and cook on High for 6 hours.

3. Divide the mix between plates and serve right away.

Nutrition Info: calories 293, fat 13.2, fiber 9.7, carbs 15.7, protein 14.3

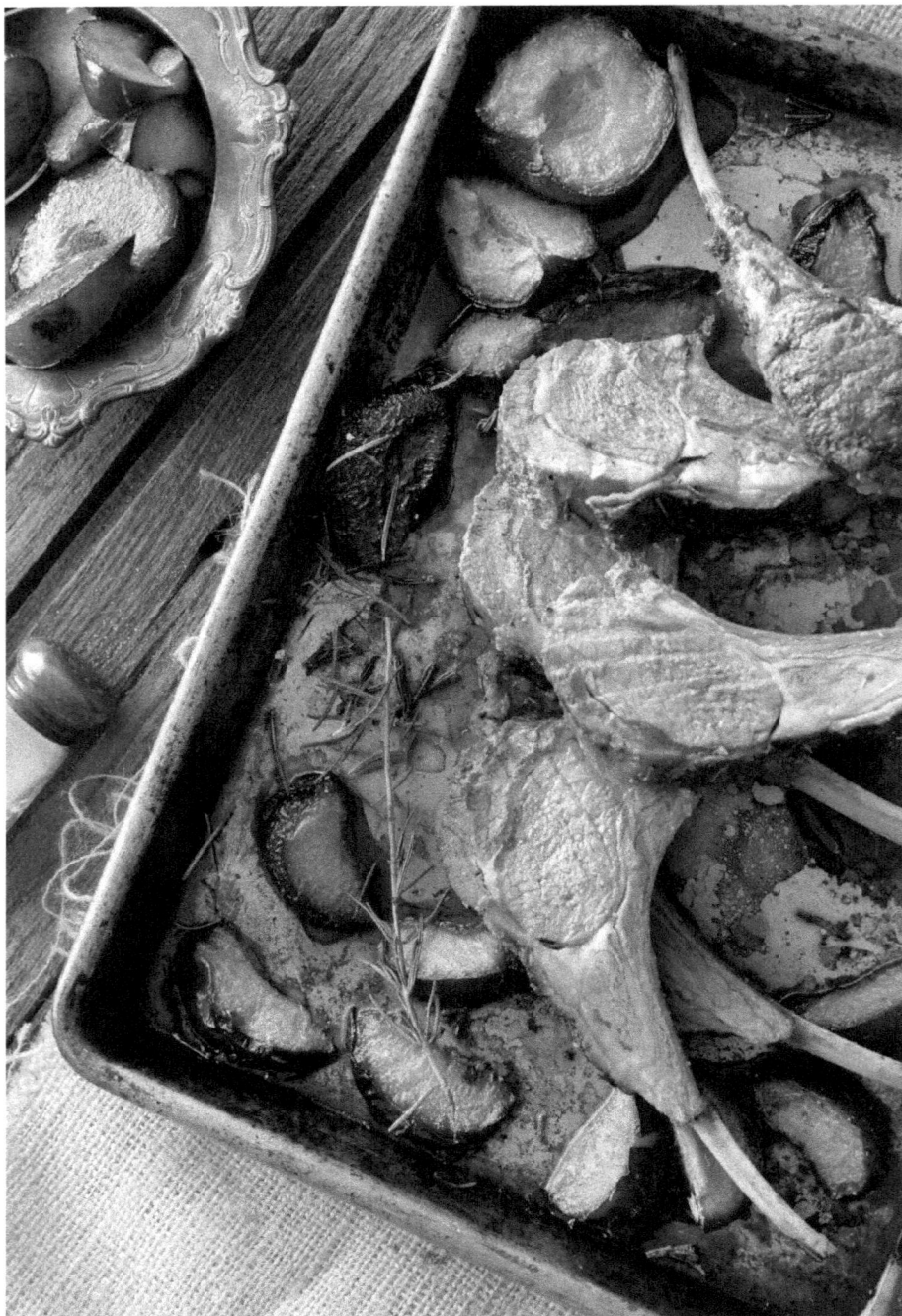

Lamb And Mango Sauce

Servings: 4
Cooking Time: 1 Hour

Ingredients:

- 2 cups Greek yogurt
- 1 cup mango, peeled and cubed
- 1 yellow onion, chopped
- 1/3 cup parsley, chopped
- 1 pound lamb, cubed
- ½ teaspoon red pepper flakes
- Salt and black pepper to the taste
- 2 tablespoons olive oil
- ¼ teaspoon cinnamon powder

Directions:
1. Heat up a pan with the oil over medium-high heat, add the meat and brown for 5 minutes.
2. Add the onion and sauté for 5 minutes more.
3. Add the rest of the ingredients, toss, bring to a simmer and cook over medium heat for 45 minutes.
4. Divide everything between plates and serve.

Nutrition Info: calories 300, fat 15.5, fiber 9.1, carbs 15.7, protein 15.5

Pork Chops And Cherries Mix

Servings: 4
Cooking Time: 12 Minutes

Ingredients:
- 4 pork chops, boneless
- Salt and black pepper to the taste
- ½ cup cranberry juice
- 1 and ½ teaspoons spicy mustard
- ½ cup dark cherries, pitted and halved
- Cooking spray

Directions:
1. Heat up a pan greased with the cooking spray over medium-high heat, add the pork chops, cook them for 5 minutes on each side and divide between plates.
2. Heat up the same pan over medium heat, add the cranberry juice and the rest of the ingredients, whisk, bring to a simmer, cook for 2 minutes, drizzle over the pork chops and serve.

Nutrition Info: calories 262, fat 8, fiber 1, carbs 16, protein 30

Lamb And Barley Mix

Servings: 4

Cooking Time: 8 Hours And 10 Minutes

Ingredients:

- 2 tablespoons olive oil
- 1 cup barley soaked overnight, drained and rinsed
- 1 pound lamb meat, cubed
- 1 red onion, chopped
- 4 garlic cloves, minced
- 3 carrots, chopped
- 6 tablespoons dill, chopped
- 2 tablespoons tomato paste
- 3 cups veggie stock
- A pinch of salt and black pepper

Directions:

1. Heat up a pan with the oil over medium-high heat, add the meat, brown for 5 minutes on each side and transfer to your slow cooker.

2. Add the barley and the rest of the ingredients, put the lid on and cook on Low for 8 hours.

3. Divide everything between plates and serve.

Nutrition Info: calories 292, fat 12.1, fiber 8.7, carbs 16.7, protein 7.2

Cashew Beef Stir Fry

Servings: 8
Cooking Time: 15 Minutes

Ingredients:

- ¼ cup coconut aminos
- 1 ½ pound ground beef
- 1 cup raw cashews
- 1 green bell pepper, julienned
- 1 red bell pepper, julienned
- 1 small can water chestnut, sliced
- 1 small onion, sliced
- 1 tablespoon garlic, minced
- 2 tablespoon ginger, grated
- 2 teaspoon coconut oil
- Salt and pepper to taste

Directions:
1. Heat a skillet over medium heat then add raw cashews. Toast for a couple of minutes or until slightly brown. Set aside.
2. In the same skillet, add the coconut oil and sauté the ground beef for 5 minutes or until brown.
3. Add the garlic, ginger and season with coconut aminos. Stir for one minute before adding the onions, bell peppers and water chestnuts. Cook until the vegetables are almost soft.

4. Season with salt and pepper to taste.

5. Add the toasted cashews last.

Nutrition Info: Calories per Serving: 324.8; Carbs: 12.4g; Protein: 19.3g; Fat: 22.0g

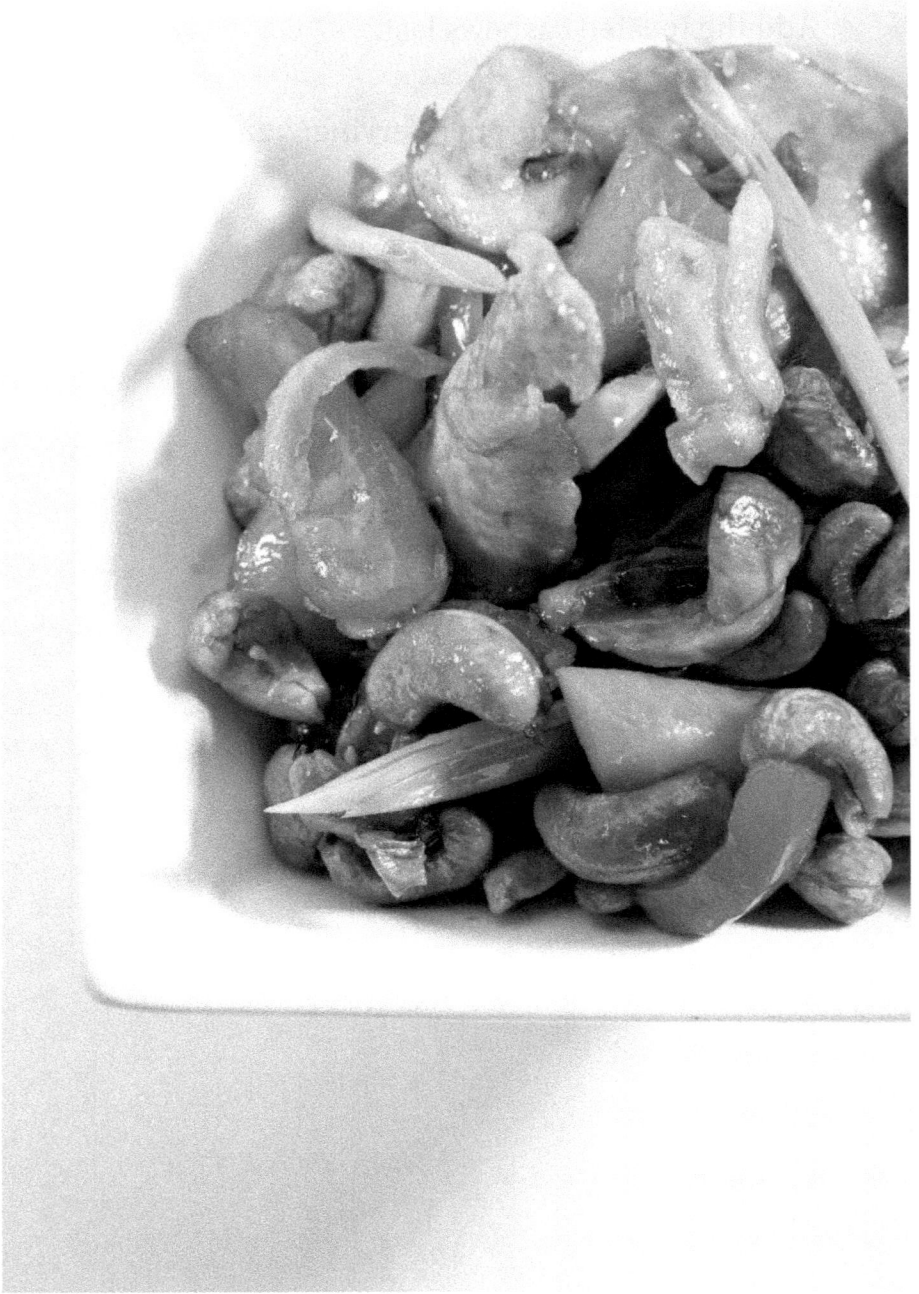

Cheesy Meat Bake

Servings: 4
Cooking Time: 40 Minutes

Ingredients:
- 6 oz pork butt, chopped
- 3 oz veal stew meat, chopped
- 1 potato, peeled
- ¼ cup cauliflower, shredded
- ¼ cup carrot, grated
- 1 teaspoon tomato paste
- 2 oz Provolone cheese, grated
- ¼ cup cream
- 1 teaspoon butter
- 1 teaspoon salt
- ½ teaspoon chili flakes

Directions:
1. Melt butter in the saucepan and add all meat.
2. Sprinkle it with salt, chili flakes, and carrot.
3. Mix up well and cook for 10 minutes.
4. Then add tomato paste and mix up well.
5. Add shredded cauliflower and roughly chopped potato.
6. Then add cream and top it with cheese.
7. Cover the saucepan with foil and transfer it in the preheated to the 365F oven.

8. Bake the casserole for 30 minutes.

Nutrition Info:Per Serving:calories 211, fat 9, fiber 1.3, carbs 9.5, protein 22.4

Shrimp And Vegetable Rice

Servings: 1 Cup
Cooking Time: 48 Minutes

Ingredients:
- 3 TB. extra-virgin olive oil
- 1 medium yellow onion, finely chopped
- 1 TB. minced garlic
- 1 cup green peas
- 2 medium carrots, shredded (1 cup)
- 4 cups water
- 2 tsp. salt
- 10 strands saffron
- 1 tsp. turmeric
- 1/2 tsp. black pepper
- 2 cups brown rice

Directions:
1. 1/2 lb. medium raw shrimp (18 to 20), shells and veins removed
2. In a large, 3-quart pot over medium heat, heat extra-virgin olive oil. Add yellow onion, and cook for 5 minutes.
3. Add garlic, green peas, and carrots, and cook for 3 minutes.
4. Add water, salt, saffron, turmeric, and black pepper; bring to a boil; and cook for about 3 minutes.

5. Add brown rice, cover, reduce heat to low, and cook for 30 minutes.

6. Gently fold shrimp into rice, cover, and cook for 10 minutes.

7. Remove from heat, fluff with a fork, cover, and set aside for 10 minutes. Serve warm.

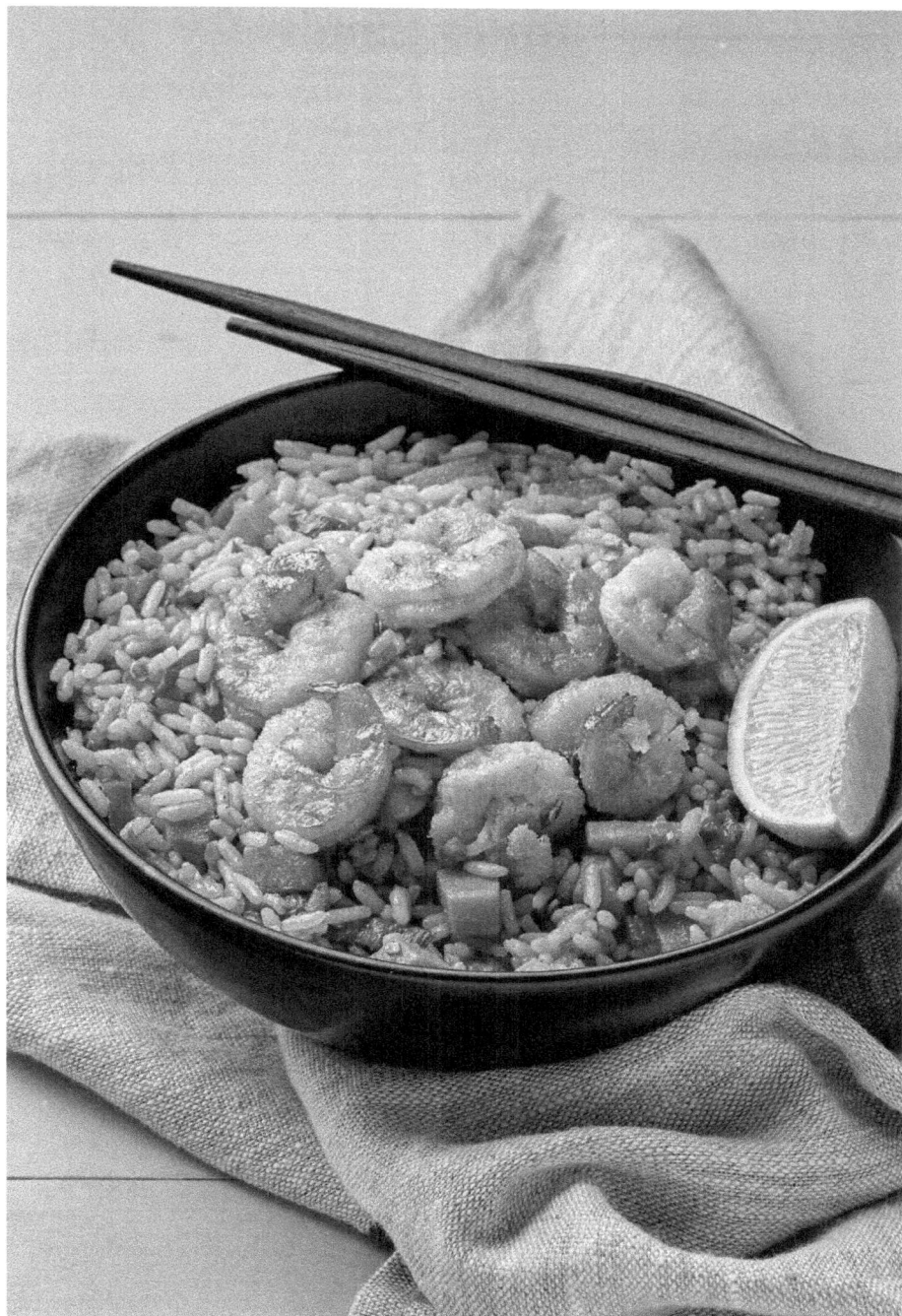

Nutmeg Lamb Mix

Servings: 6
Cooking Time: 30 Minutes

Ingredients:

- 1 red onion, chopped
- 1 tablespoon olive oil
- 1 garlic clove, minced
- 1 pound lamb meat, cubed
- ¾ cup celery, chopped
- Salt and black pepper to the taste
- 29 ounces canned tomatoes, drained and chopped
- 1 cup veggie stock
- ½ teaspoon nutmeg, ground
- 2 teaspoons parsley, chopped

Directions:

1. Heat up a pan with the oil over medium heat, add the onion and the garlic and sauté for 5 minutes.
2. Add the meat and brown for 5 minutes more.
3. Add the rest of the ingredients, bring to a simmer and cook over medium heat for 20 minutes.
4. Divide everything between plates and serve.

Nutrition Info: calories 284, fat 13.3, fiber 8.2, carbs 14.5, protein 17.6

Lamb And Zucchini Mix

Servings: 4

Cooking Time: 4 Hours

Ingredients:

- 2 pounds lamb stew meat, cubed
- 1 and ½ tablespoons avocado oil
- 3 zucchinis, sliced
- 1 brown onion, chopped
- 3 garlic cloves, minced
- 1 tablespoon thyme, dried
- 2 teaspoons sage, dried
- 1 cup chicken stock
- 2 tablespoons tomato paste

Directions:

1. In a slow cooker, combine the lamb with the oil, zucchinis and the rest of the ingredients, toss, put the lid on and cook on High for 4 hours.
 2. Divide the mix between plates and serve right away.

Nutrition Info: calories 272, fat 14.5, fiber 10.1, carbs 20.3, protein 13.3

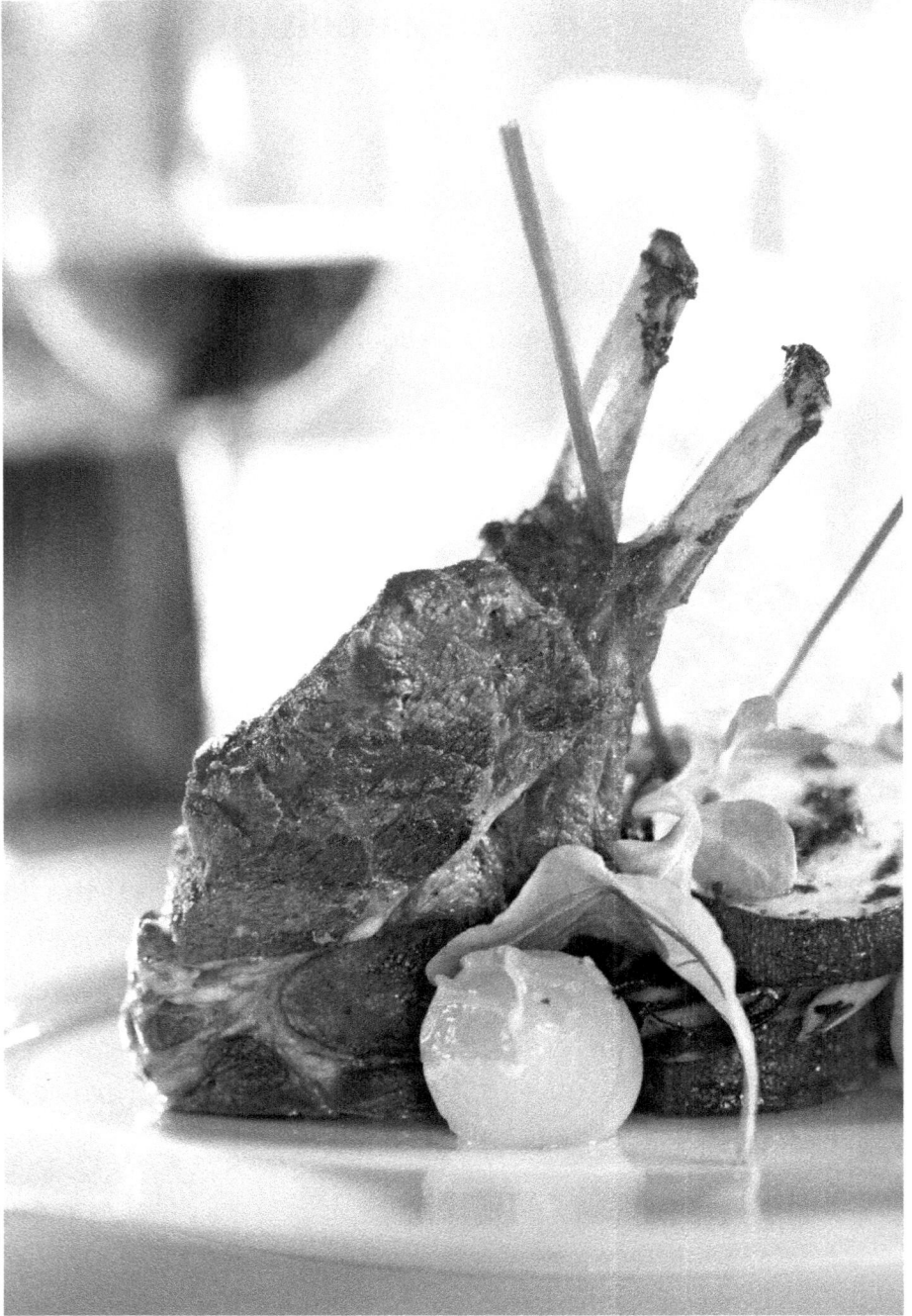

Pork And Green Beans Mix

Servings: 5
Cooking Time: 35 Minutes

Ingredients:
- 1 cup ground pork
- 1 sweet pepper, chopped
- 1 oz green beans, chopped
- ½ onion, sliced
- 2 oz Parmesan, grated
- ¼ cup chicken stock
- 1 teaspoon olive oil
- ½ teaspoon cayenne pepper
- 1 teaspoon dried oregano
- ½ teaspoon dried basil
- 1 teaspoon paprika
- ½ cup crushed tomatoes, canned

Directions:
1. Pour olive oil in the saucepan and heat it up.
2. Add ground pork and cook it for 2 minutes.
3. Then stir it carefully and sprinkle with cayenne pepper, dried oregano, dried basil, and paprika.
4. Roast the meat for 5 minutes more and add green beans, sweet pepper, and sliced onion.
5. Add chicken stock and crushed tomatoes.
6. Mix up the ground pork and close the lid.

7. Cook the meal for 20 minutes over the medium heat. Stir it from time to time.

8. Then sprinkle the bolognese meat with Parmesan and mix up well. 9. Cook the meal for 5 minutes more.

Nutrition Info:Per Serving:calories 257, fat 16.6, fiber 1.9, carbs 6.2, protein 20.9

Artichoke Beef Roast

Servings: 6
Cooking Time: 45 Minutes

Ingredients:
- 2 lbs beef roast, cubed
- 1 tbsp garlic, minced
- 1 onion, chopped
- 1/2 tsp paprika
- 1 tbsp parsley, chopped
- 2 tomatoes, chopped
- 1 tbsp capers, chopped
- 10 oz can artichokes, drained and chopped
- 2 cups chicken stock
- 1 tbsp olive oil
- Pepper
- Salt

Directions:
1. Add oil into the instant pot and set the pot on sauté mode.
2. Add garlic and onion and sauté for 5 minutes.
3. Add meat and cook until brown.
4. Add remaining ingredients and stir well.
5. Seal pot with lid and cook on high for 35 minutes.
6. Once done, allow to release pressure naturally. Remove lid.

7. Serve and enjoy.

Nutrition Info: Calories 344 Fat 12.2 g Carbohydrates 9.2 g Sugar 2.6 g Protein 48.4 g Cholesterol 135 mg

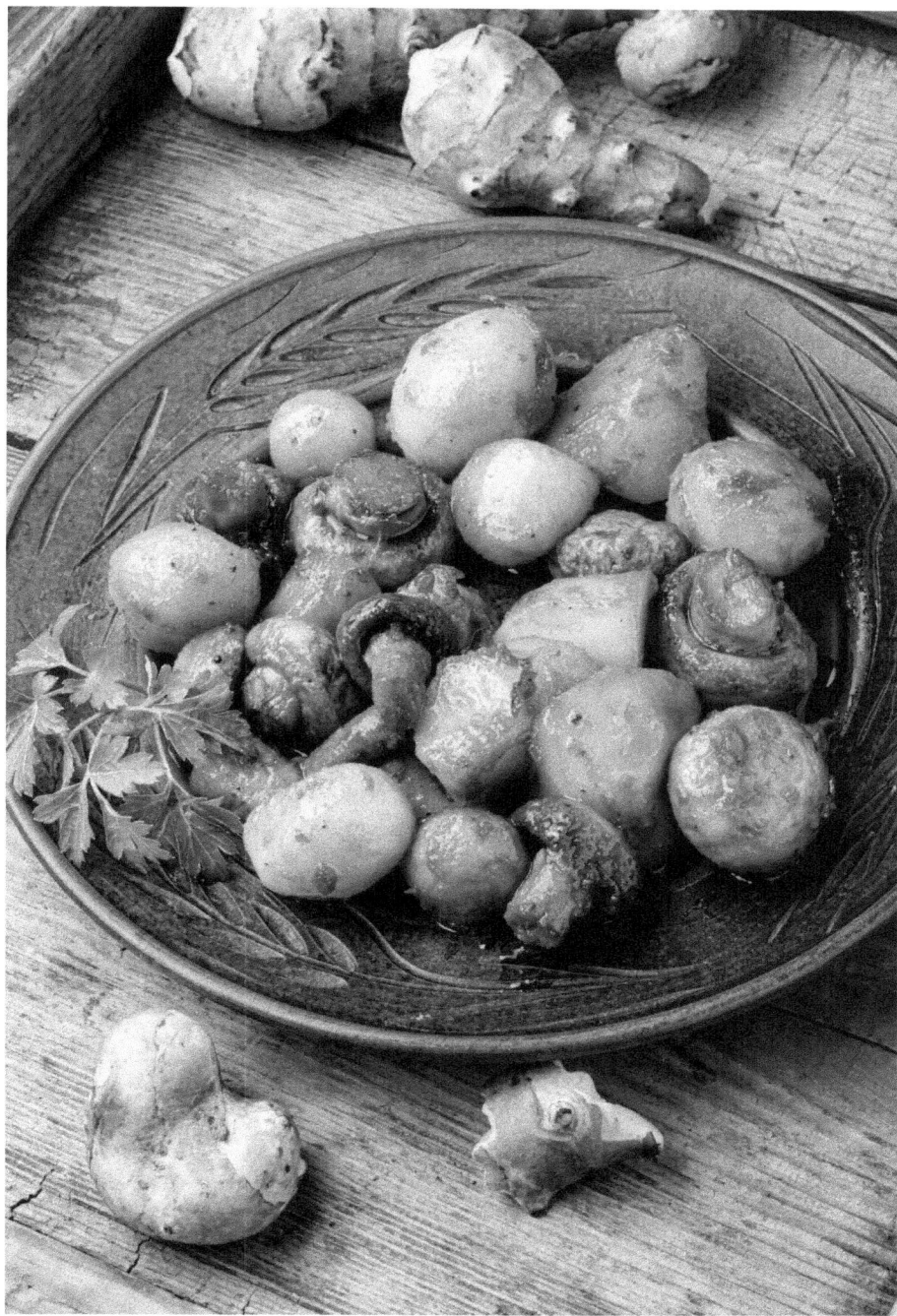

Oregano And Pesto Lamb

Servings: 4
Cooking Time: 25 Minutes

Ingredients:
- 2 pounds pork shoulder, boneless and cubed
- ¼ cup olive oil
- 2 teaspoons oregano, dried
- ¼ cup lemon juice
- 3 garlic cloves, minced
- 2 teaspoons basil pesto
- Salt and black pepper to the taste

Directions:
1. Heat up a pan with the oil over medium-high heat, add the pork and brown for 5 minutes.
2. Add the rest of the ingredients, cook for 20 minutes more, tossing the mix from time to time, divide between plates and serve.

Nutrition Info: calories 297, fat 14.5, fiber 9.3, carbs 16.8, protein 22.2

Italian Beef Roast

Servings: 6
Cooking Time: 50 Minutes

Ingredients:
- 2 1/2 lbs beef roast, cut into chunks
- 1 cup chicken broth
- 1 cup red wine
- 2 tbsp Italian seasoning
- 2 tbsp olive oil
- 1 bell pepper, chopped
- 2 celery stalks, chopped
- 1 tsp garlic, minced
- 1 onion, sliced
- Pepper
- Salt

Directions:
1. Add oil into the instant pot and set the pot on sauté mode.
2. Add the meat into the pot and sauté until brown.
3. Add onion, bell pepper, and celery and sauté for 5 minutes.
4. Add remaining ingredients and stir well.
5. Seal pot with lid and cook on high for 40 minutes.
6. Once done, allow to release pressure naturally. Remove lid.

7. Stir well and serve.

Nutrition Info: Calories 460 Fat 18.2 g Carbohydrates 5.3 g Sugar 2.7 g Protein 58.7 g Cholesterol 172 mg

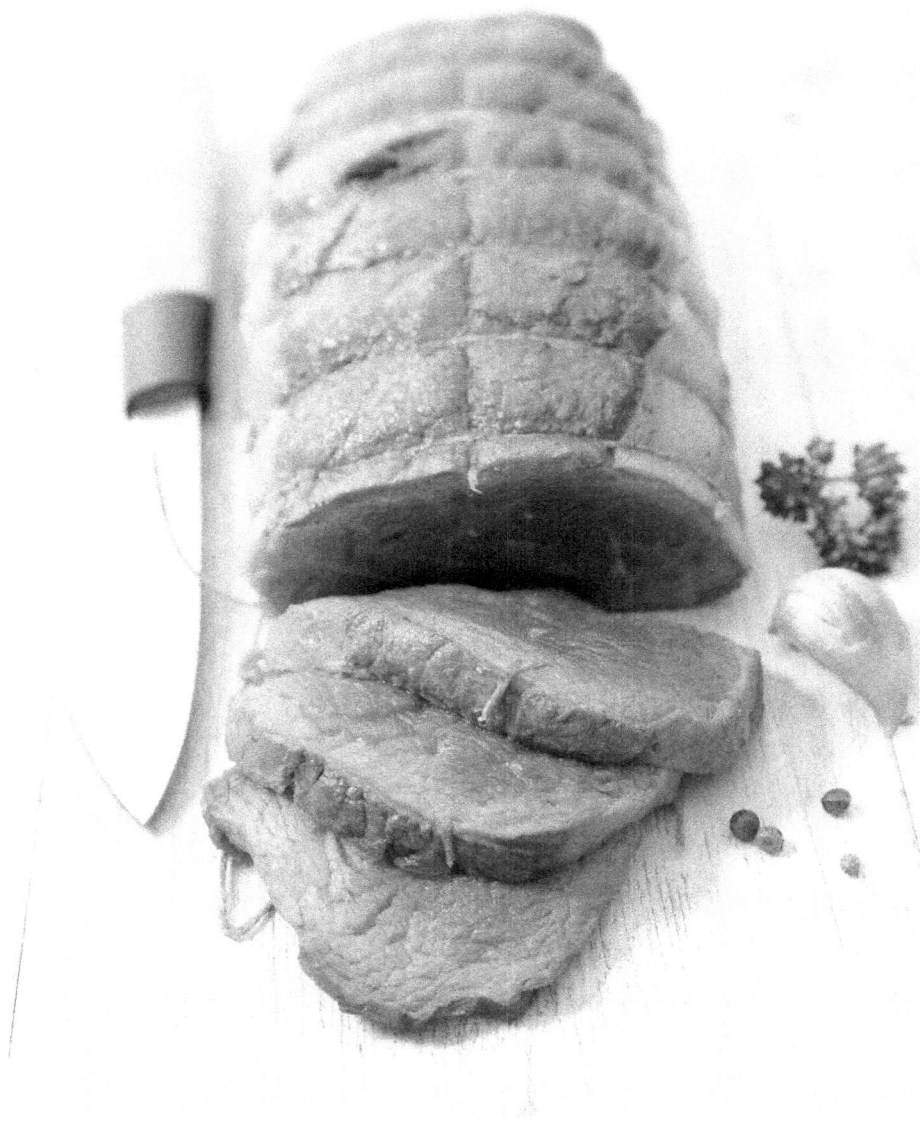

Chili Pork Meatballs

Servings: 4
Cooking Time: 20 Minutes

Ingredients:
- 1 pound pork meat, ground
- ½ cup parsley, chopped
- 1 cup yellow onion, chopped
- 4 garlic cloves, minced
- 1 tablespoon ginger, grated
- 1 Thai chili, chopped
- 2 tablespoons olive oil
- 1 cup veggie stock
- 2 tablespoons sweet paprika

Directions:
1. In a bowl, mix the pork with the other ingredients except the oil, stock and paprika, stir well and shape medium meatballs out of this mix.
2. Heat up a pan with the oil over medium-high heat, add the meatballs and cook for 4 minutes on each side.
3. Add the stock and the paprika, toss gently, simmer everything over medium heat for 12 minutes more, divide into bowls and serve.

Nutrition Info: calories 224, fat 18, fiber 9.3, carbs 11.5, protein 14.4

Worcestershire Pork Chops

Servings: 3
Cooking Time: 15 Minutes

Ingredients:
2 tablespoons Worcestershire sauce
8 oz pork loin chops
1 tablespoon lemon juice
1 teaspoon olive oil

Directions:
1. Mix up together Worcestershire sauce, lemon juice, and olive oil.
2. Brush the pork loin chops with the sauce mixture from each side.
3. Preheat the grill to 395F.
4. Place the pork chops in the grill and cook them for 5 minutes.
5. Then flip the pork chops on another side and brush with remaining sauce mixture.
6. Grill the meat for 7-8 minutes more.

Nutrition Info:Per Serving:calories 267, fat 20.4, fiber 0, carbs 2.1, protein 17 249.

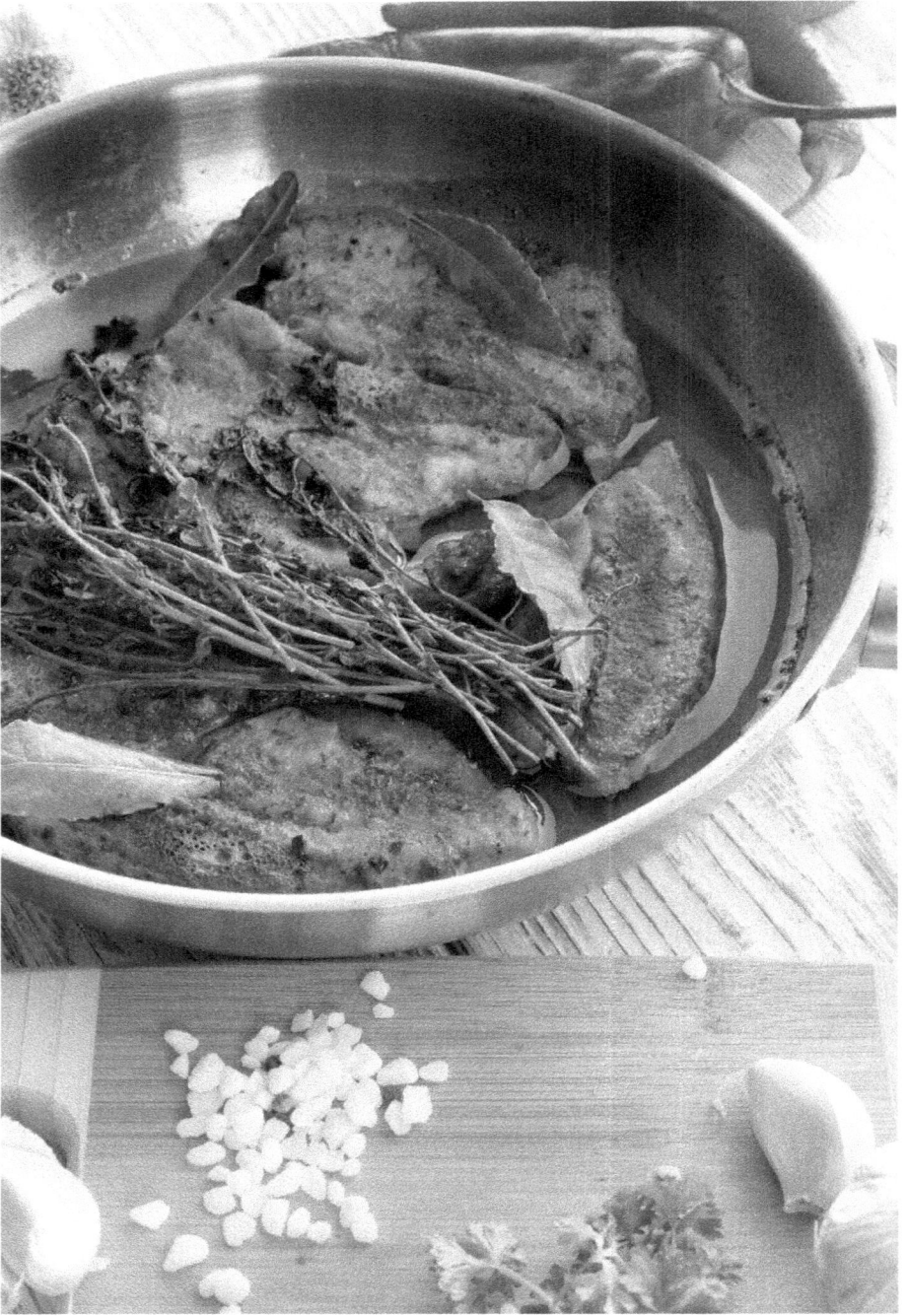

Sage Tomato Beef

Servings: 4
Cooking Time: 40 Minutes

Ingredients:
- 2 lbs beef stew meat, cubed
- 1/4 cup tomato paste
- 1 tsp garlic, minced
- 2 cups chicken stock
- 1 onion, chopped
- 2 tbsp olive oil
- 1 tbsp sage, chopped
- Pepper
- Salt

Directions:
1. Add oil into the instant pot and set the pot on sauté mode.
2. Add garlic and onion and sauté for 5 minutes.
3. Add meat and sauté for 5 minutes.
4. Add remaining ingredients and stir well.
5. Seal pot with lid and cook on high for 30 minutes.
6. Once done, allow to release pressure naturally. Remove lid. 7. Serve and enjoy.

Nutrition Info: Calories 515 Fat 21.5 g Carbohydrates 7 g Sugar 3.6 g Protein 70 g Cholesterol 203 mg

Square Meat Pies (sfeeha)

Servings: 1 Meat Pie

Cooking Time: 20 Minutes

Ingredients:
- 1 large yellow onion
- 2 large tomatoes
- 1 lb. ground beef
- 11/4 tsp. salt
- 1/2 tsp. ground black pepper
- 1 tsp. seven spices
- 1 batch Multipurpose Dough (recipe in Chapter 12)

Directions:

1. Preheat the oven to 425°F.

2. In a food processor fitted with a chopping blade, pulse yellow onion and tomatoes for 30 seconds.

3. Transfer tomato-onion mixture to a large bowl. Add beef, salt, black pepper, and seven spices, and mix well.

4. Form Multipurpose Dough into 18 balls, and roll out to 4-inch circles.

Spoon 2 tablespoons meat mixture onto center of each dough circle. Pinch together the two opposite sides of dough up to meat mixture, and pinch the opposite two sides together, forming a square. Place meat pies on a baking sheet, and bake for 20 minutes.

5. Serve warm or at room temperature.

Lamb And Wine Sauce

Servings: 4

Cooking Time: 2 Hours And 40 Minutes

Ingredients:

- 2 tablespoons olive oil
- 2 pounds leg of lamb, trimmed and sliced
- 3 garlic cloves, chopped
- 2 yellow onions, chopped
- 3 cups veggie stock
- 2 cups dry red wine
- 2 tablespoons tomato paste
- 4 tablespoons avocado oil
- 1 teaspoon thyme, chopped
- Salt and black pepper to the taste

Directions:

1. Heat up a pan with the oil over medium-high heat, add the meat, brown for 5 minutes on each side and transfer to a roasting pan.

2. Heat up the pan again over medium heat, add the avocado oil, add the onions and garlic and sauté for 5 minutes.

3. Add the remaining ingredients, stir, bring to a simmer and cook for 10 minutes.

4. Pour the sauce over the meat, introduce the pan in the oven and bake at 370 degrees F for 2 hours and 20 minutes.

5. Divide everything between plates and serve.

Nutrition Info: calories 273, fat 21, fiber 11.1, carbs 16.2, protein 18.3

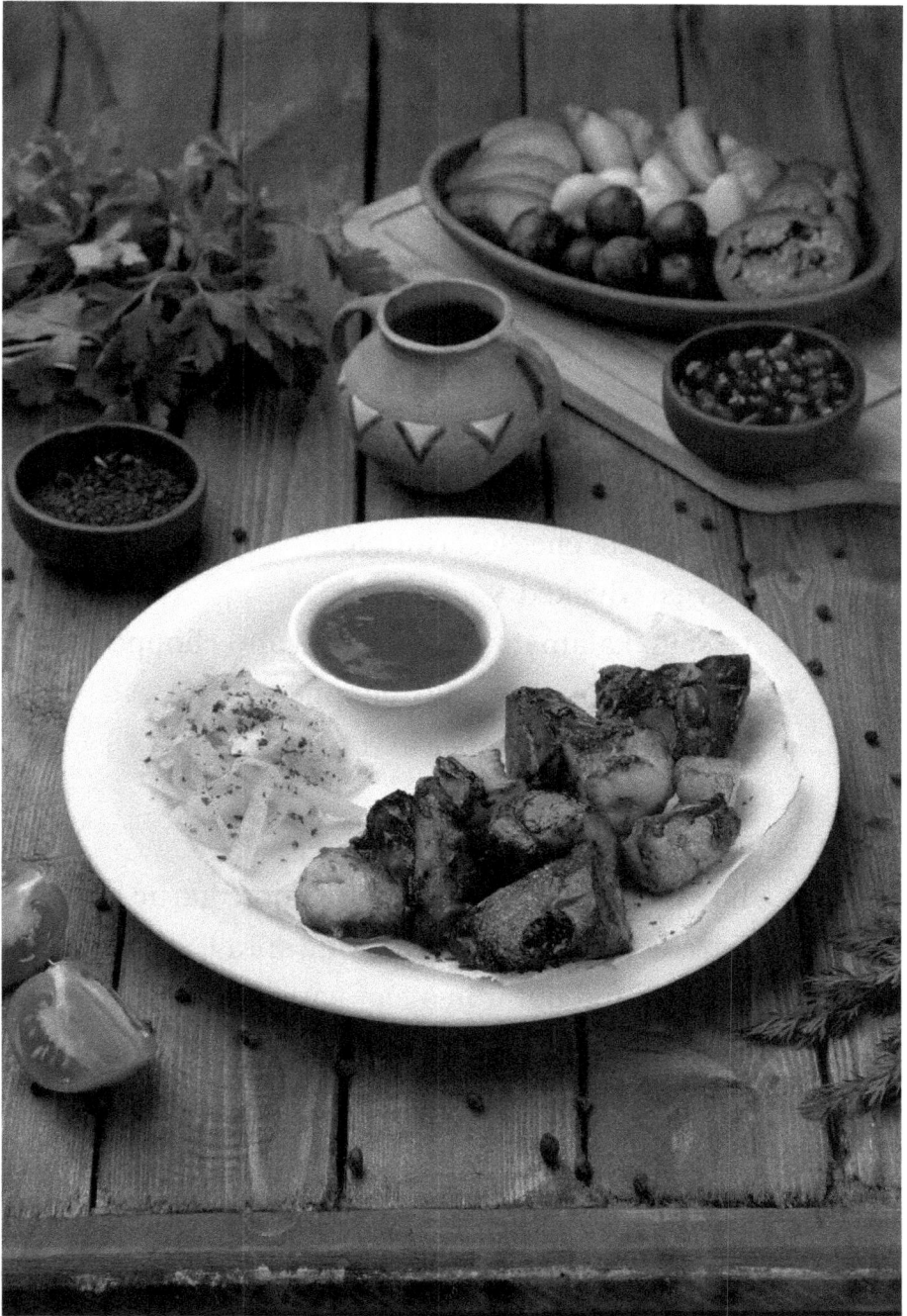

Pork Meatloaf

Servings: 6

Cooking Time: 1 Hour And 20 Minutes

Ingredients:
- 1 red onion, chopped
- Cooking spray
- 2 garlic cloves, minced
- 2 pounds pork stew, ground
- 1 cup almond milk
- ¼ cup feta cheese, crumbled
- 2 eggs, whisked
- 1/3 cup kalamata olives, pitted and chopped
- 4 tablespoons oregano, chopped
- Salt and black pepper to the taste

Directions:

1. In a bowl, mix the meat with the onion, garlic and the other ingredients except the cooking spray, stir well, shape your meatloaf and put it in a loaf pan greased with cooking spray.

2. Bake the meatloaf at 370 degrees F for 1 hour and 20 minutes.

3. Serve the meatloaf warm.

Nutrition Info: calories 350, fat 23, fiber 1, carbs 17, protein 24

Lamb And Rice

Servings: 4

Cooking Time: 1 Hour And 10 Minutes

Ingredients:

- 1 tablespoon lime juice
- 1 yellow onion, chopped
- 1 pound lamb, cubed
- 1 ounce avocado oil
- 2 garlic cloves, minced
- Salt and black pepper to the taste
- 2 cups veggie stock
- 1 cup brown rice
- A handful parsley, chopped

Directions:

1. Heat up a pan with the avocado oil over medium-high heat, add the onion, stir and sauté for 5 minutes.

2. Add the meat and brown for 5 minutes more.

3. Add the rest of the ingredients except the parsley, bring to a simmer and cook over medium heat for 1 hour.

4. Add the parsley, toss, divide everything between plates and serve.

Nutrition Info: calories 302, fat 13.2, fiber 10.7, carbs 15.7, protein 14.3

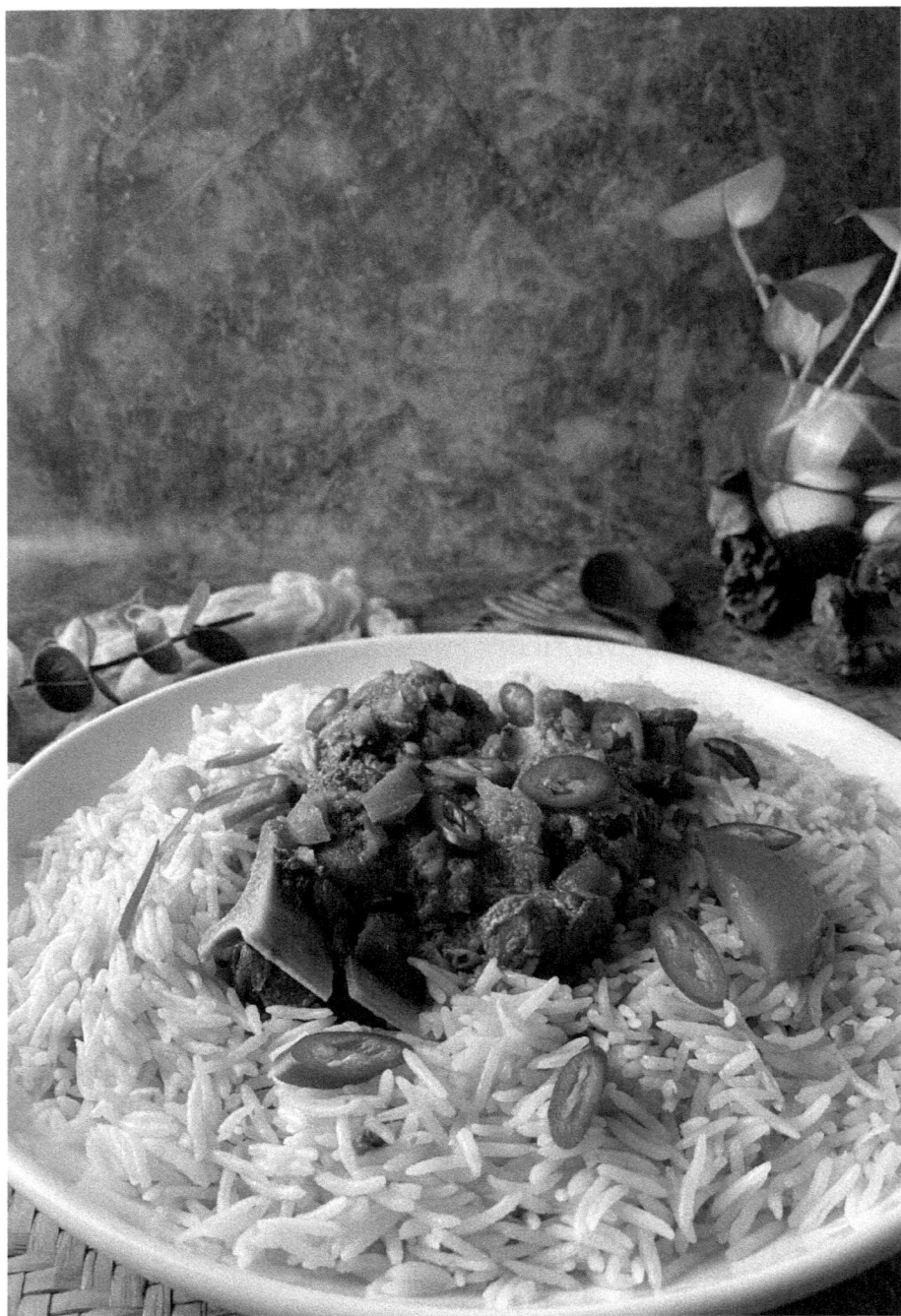

Italian Beef

Servings: 4
Cooking Time: 35 Minutes

Ingredients:
- 1 lb ground beef
- 1 tbsp olive oil
- 1/2 cup mozzarella cheese, shredded
- 1/2 cup tomato puree
- 1 tsp basil
- 1 tsp oregano
- 1/2 onion, chopped
- 1 carrot, chopped
- 14 oz can tomatoes, diced
- Pepper
- Salt

Directions:
1. Add oil into the instant pot and set the pot on sauté mode.
2. Add onion and sauté for 2 minutes.
3. Add meat and sauté until browned.
4. Add remaining ingredients except for cheese and stir well.
5. Seal pot with lid and cook on high for 35 minutes.

6. Once done, release pressure using quick release. Remove lid. 7. Add cheese and stir well and cook on sauté mode until cheese is melted. 8. Serve and enjoy.

Nutrition Info: Calories 297 Fat 11.3 g Carbohydrates 11.1 g Sugar 6.2 g Protein 37.1 g Cholesterol 103 mg

Pork Chops And Peppercorns Mix

Servings: 4

Cooking Time: 20 Minutes

Ingredients:

- 1 cup red onion, sliced
- 1 tablespoon black peppercorns, crushed
- ¼ cup veggie stock
- 5 garlic cloves, minced
- A pinch of salt and black pepper
- 2 tablespoons olive oil
- 4 pork chops

Directions:

1. Heat up a pan with the oil over medium-high heat, add the pork chops and brown for 4 minutes on each side.

2. Add the onion and the garlic and cook for 2 minutes more.

3. Add the rest of the ingredients, cook everything for 10 minutes, tossing the mix from time to time, divide between plates and serve.

Nutrition Info: calories 232, fat 9.2, fiber 5.6, carbs 13.3, protein 24.2

Pork And Tomato Meatloaf

Servings: 8
Cooking Time: 55 Minutes

Ingredients:

- 2 cups ground pork
- 1 egg, beaten
- ¼ cup crushed tomatoes
- 1 teaspoon salt
- 1 teaspoon ground black pepper
- 1 oz Swiss cheese, grated
- 1 teaspoon minced garlic
- 1/3 onion, diced
- ¼ cup black olives, chopped
- 1 jalapeno pepper, chopped
- 1 teaspoon dried basil
- Cooking spray

Directions:

1. Spray the loaf mold with cooking spray.

2. Then combine together ground pork, egg, crushed tomatoes, salt, ground black pepper. Grated Swiss cheese, minced garlic, onion, olives, jalapeno pepper, and dried basil.

3. Stir the mass until it is homogenous and transfer it in the prepared loaf mold.

4. Flatten the surface of meatloaf well and cover with foil.

5. Bake the meatloaf for 40 minutes at 375F.

6. Then discard the foil and bake the meal for 15 minutes more.

7. Chill the cooked meatloaf to the room temperature and then remove it from the loaf mold.

8. Slice it on the servings.

Nutrition Info:Per Serving:calories 265, fat 18.3, fiber 0.6, carbs 1.9, protein 22.1

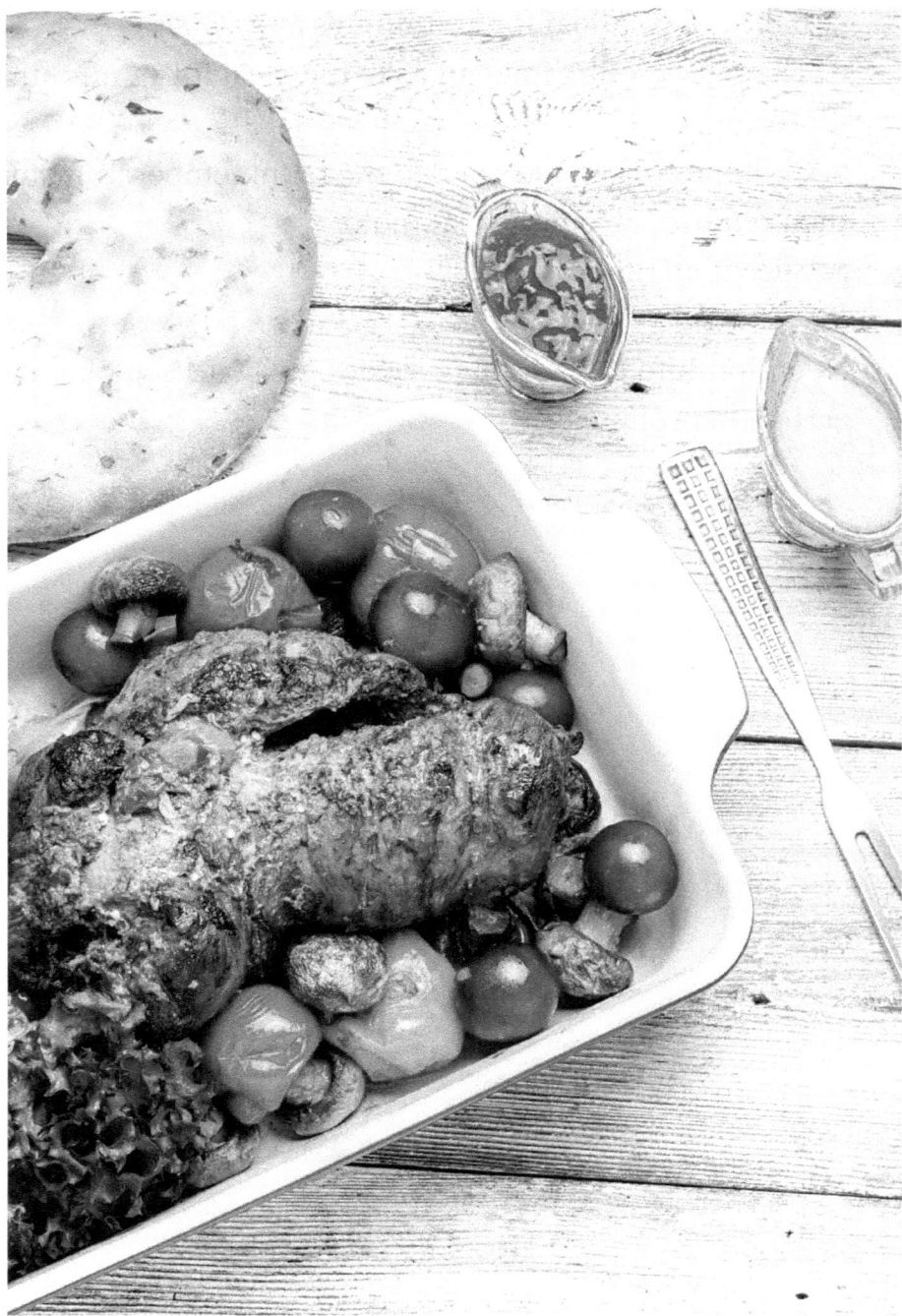

Beef And Eggplant Moussaka

Servings: 3
Cooking Time: 50 Minutes

Ingredients:

- 1 small eggplant, sliced
- 1 teaspoon olive oil
- ½ cup cream
- 1 egg, beaten
- 1 tablespoon wheat flour, whole grain
- 1 teaspoon cornstarch
- 3 oz Romano cheese, grated
- ½ cup ground beef
- ¼ teaspoon minced garlic
- 1 tablespoon Italian parsley, chopped
- 3 tablespoons tomato sauce
- ¾ teaspoon ground nutmeg

Directions:

1. Sprinkle the eggplants with olive oil and ground nutmeg and arrange in the casserole mold in one layer.
2. After this, place the ground beef in the skillet.
3. Add minced garlic, Italian parsley, and ground nutmeg.
4. Then add tomato sauce and mix up the mixture well.
5. Roast it for 10 minutes over the medium heat.
6. Make the sauce: in the saucepan whisk together cream with egg.

7. Bring the liquid to boil (simmer it constantly) and add wheat flour, cornstarch, and cheese. Stir well.

8. Bring the liquid to boil and stir till cheese is melted. Remove the sauce from the heat.

9. Put the cooked ground beef over the eggplants and flatten well.

10. Then pour the cream sauce over the ground beef.

11. Cover the meal with foil and secure the edges.

12. Bake moussaka for 30 minutes at 365F.

Nutrition Info:Per Serving:calories 271, fat 16.1, fiber 5.9, carbs 15.4, protein 17.6

Hearty Meat And Potatoes

Servings: 2 Cups

Cooking Time: 30 Minutes

Ingredients:

- 1 lb. ground beef or lamb
- 1/4 cup extra-virgin olive oil
- 1 large yellow onion, chopped
- 5 large potatoes, peeled and cubed
- 11/2 tsp. salt
- 1 TB. seven spices
- 1/2 tsp. ground black pepper

Directions:

1. In a large, 3-quart pot over medium heat, brown beef for 5 minutes, breaking up chunks with a wooden spoon.
2. Add extra-virgin olive oil and yellow onion, and cook for 5 minutes.
3. Toss in potatoes, salt, seven spices, and black pepper. Cover and cook for 10 minutes. Toss gently, and cook for 10 more minutes.
4. Serve warm with a side of Greek yogurt.

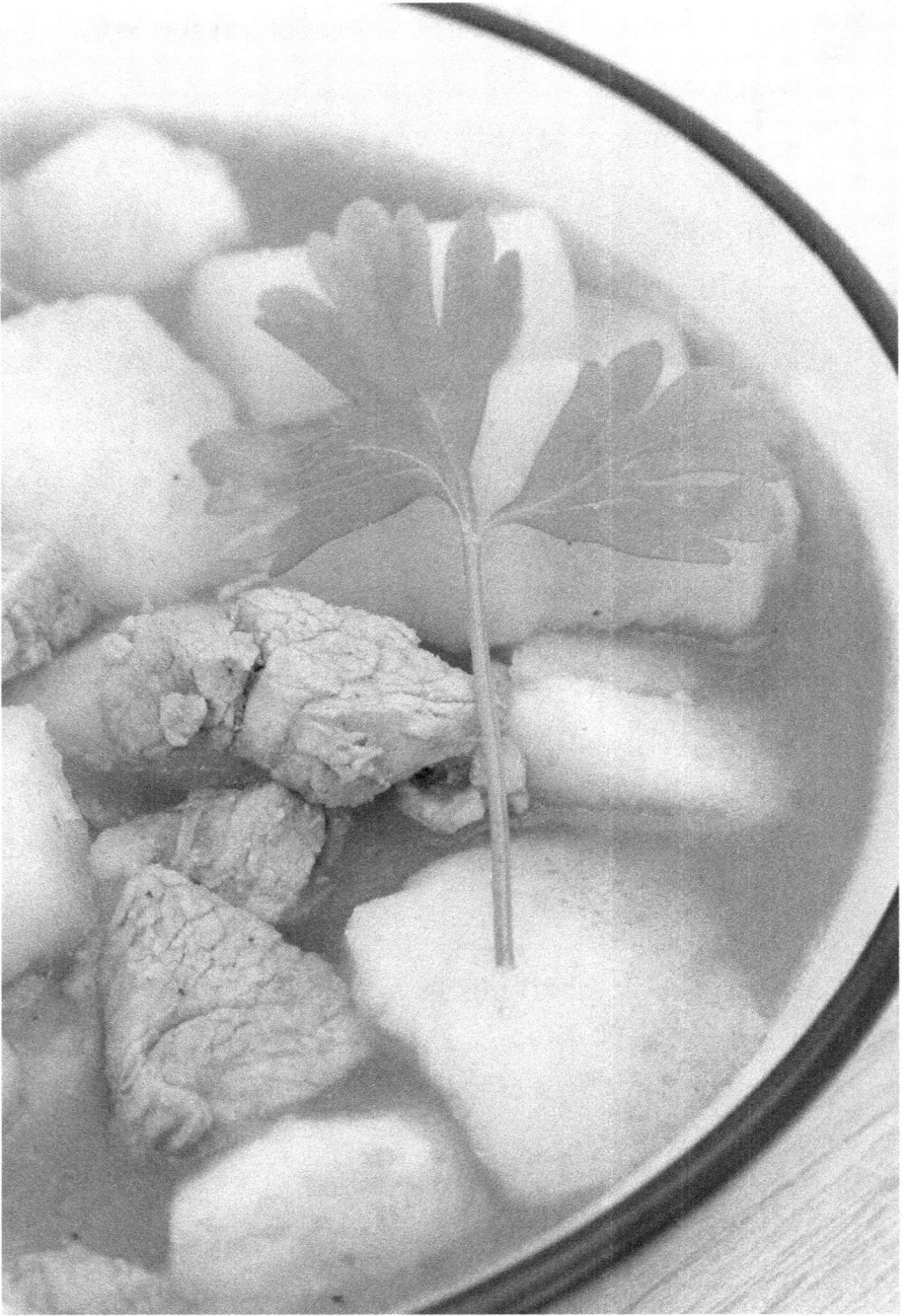

Pita Sandwiches

Servings: 1 Pita Sandwich

Cooking Time: 20 Minutes

Ingredients:
- 1 lb. ground beef
- 1 tsp. salt
- 1/2 tsp. ground black pepper
- 1 tsp. seven spices
- 4 (6- or 7-in.) pitas

Directions:

1. Preheat the oven to 400°F.

2. In a medium bowl, combine beef, salt, black pepper, and seven spices.

3. Lay out pitas on the counter, and divide beef mixture evenly among them, and spread beef to edge of pitas.

4. Place pitas on a baking sheet, and bake for 20 minutes.

5. Serve warm with Greek yogurt.

Easy Chicken With Capers Skillet

Servings: 4

Cooking Time: 35 Minutes

Ingredients:

- 4 boneless skinless chicken breast halves (6 ounces each)
- 1/4 teaspoon salt
- 1/4 teaspoon pepper
- 3 tablespoons olive oil
- 1-pint grape tomatoes
- 16 pitted Greek or ripe olives, sliced
- 3 tablespoons capers, drained

Directions:

1. Place a cast iron skillet on medium high fire and heat for 5 minutes.

2. Meanwhile, season chicken with pepper and salt.

3. Add oil to pan and heat for another minute. Add chicken and increase fire to high. Brown sides for 4 minutes per side.

4. Lower fire to medium and add capers and tomatoes.

5. Bake uncovered in a 475oF preheated oven for 12 minutes. 6. Remove from oven and let it sit for 5 minutes before serving.

Nutrition Info: Calories per Serving: 336; Carbs: 6.0g; Protein: 36.0g; Fats: 18.0g

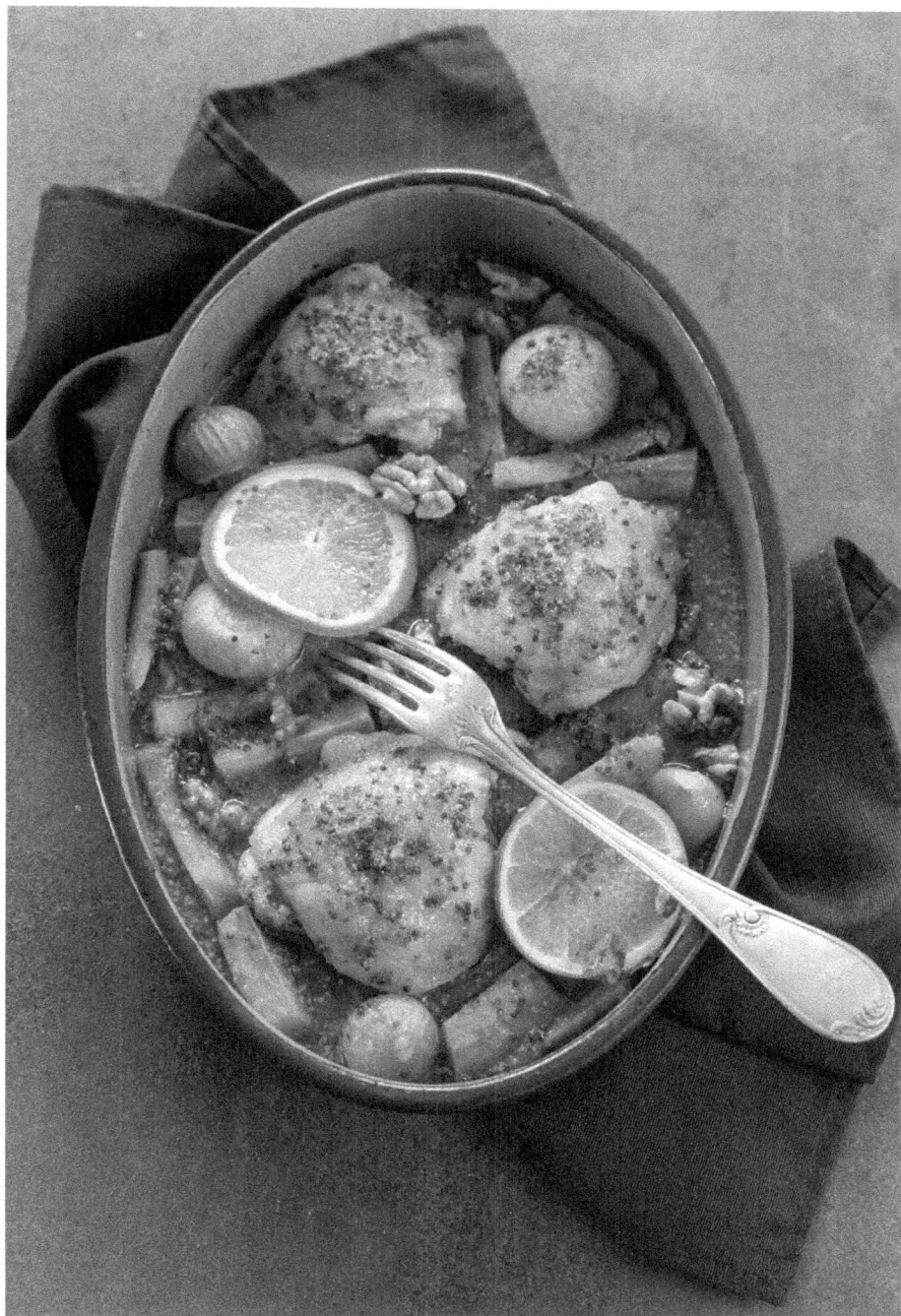

Lamb And Dill Apples

Servings: 4

Cooking Time: 25 Minutes

Ingredients:

- 3 green apples, cored, peeled and cubed
- Juice of 1 lemon
- 1 pound lamb stew meat, cubed
- 1 small bunch dill, chopped
- 3 ounces heavy cream
- 2 tablespoon olive oil
- Salt and black pepper to the taste

Directions:

1. Heat up a pan with the oil over medium-high heat, add the lamb and brown for 5 minutes.

2. Add the rest of the ingredients, bring to a simmer and cook over medium heat for 20 minutes.

3. Divide the mix between plates and serve.

Nutrition Info: calories 328, fat 16.7, fiber 10.5, carbs 21.6, protein 14.7

Tomatoes And Carrots Pork Mix

Servings: 4

Cooking Time: 7 Hours

Ingredients:
- 2 tablespoons olive oil
- ½ cup chicken stock
- 1 tablespoon ginger, grated
- Salt and black pepper to the taste
- 2 and ½ pounds pork stew meat, roughly cubed
- 2 cups tomatoes, chopped
- 4 ounces carrots, chopped
- 1 tablespoon cilantro, chopped

Directions:

1. In your slow cooker, combine the oil with the stock, ginger and the rest of the ingredients, put the lid on and cook on Low for 7 hours.

2. Divide the mix between plates and serve.

Nutrition Info: calories 303, fat 15, fiber 8.6, carbs 14.9, protein 10.8

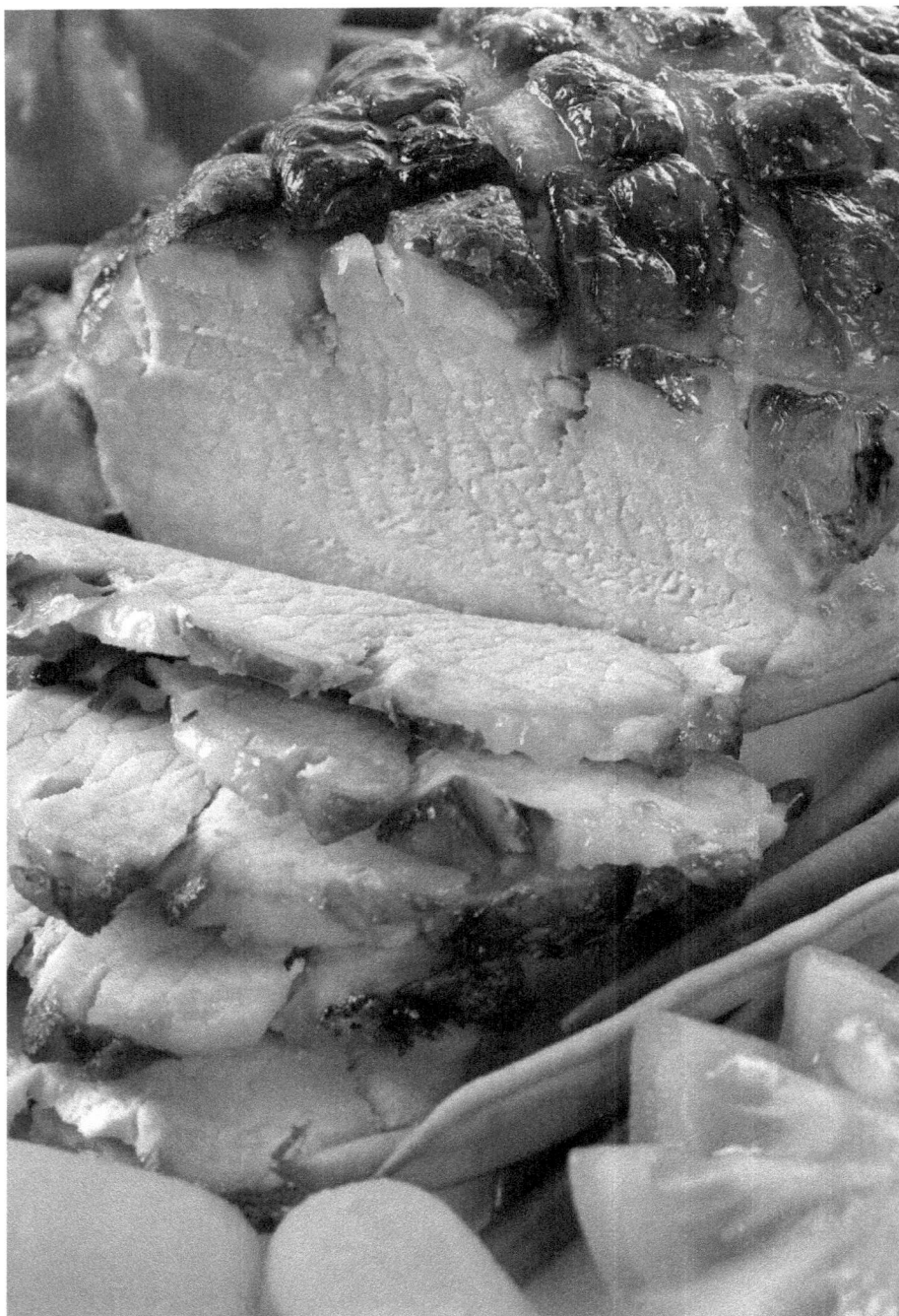

Rosemary Pork Chops

Servings: 4

Cooking Time: 35 Minutes

Ingredients:

- 4 pork loin chops, boneless
- Salt and black pepper to the taste
- 4 garlic cloves, minced
- 1 tablespoon rosemary, chopped
- 1 tablespoon olive oil

Directions:

1. In a roasting pan, combine the pork chops with the rest of the ingredients, toss, and bake at 425 degrees F for 10 minutes.

2. Reduce the heat to 350 degrees F and cook the chops for 25 minutes more.

3. Divide the chops between plates and serve with a side salad.

Nutrition Info: calories 161, fat 5, fiber 1, carbs 1, protein 25

Notes